Miller's exemplary journey through her husband's diagnosis and illness is inspirational and of benefit to anyone who has a loved one diagnosed with Alzheimer's disease. For those not fortunate enough to hear this outstanding speaker read her poetry, this collection of poems is the next best thing.

—Jan Mashman, M.D.
Associated Neurologists, Danbury, CT, retired

Every now and then a book comes along that tugs at your heart, touches your soul, and could very well be your own story. That book is here and addresses the sorrows and successes inherent in this horrible disease that all caregivers grapple with. Anyone touched by Alzheimer's needs My Life Rearranged.

—Lana Wallace

You spoke my thoughts, my feelings, and my yearnings at losing my spirit. Your book is the first piece of literature that pierced my heart. I have never seen a more unclouded picture of life with a beloved partner who becomes a stranger.

—Gloria Gutnes

I was finally able to read you book and once I started reading it, I had trouble putting it down. You have written a beautiful, simple, yet profound book. It is so honest it almost took my breath away.

—Francine Nuenen

My Life Rearranged is an incredible recollection of Susan's journey that provides insight, knowledge, and issues that all caregivers can relate to and learn from. A must-have.

—Susan's Support Group members

My Life

Life

Rearranged

Musings of
an Alzheimer
Caregiver

Susan G. Miller

My Life Rearranged: Musings of an Alzheimer's Caregiver
Susan G. Miller

Cover, Interior design and eBook conversion:
Rebecca Finkel, F + P Graphic Design, FPGD.com
Editing: Peggie Ireland
Book consulting: Judith Briles, The Book Shepherd, TheBookShepherd.com

Library of Congress Catalog Number: data on file
Health | Geriatrics | Dementia | Alzheimer's

ISBN paper 978-0967958408
ISBN eBook   978-0967958415

Printed in the USA

Imagine *coming home from the store and laying your package down, only to find it gone thirty minutes later, nowhere to be found.*

Imagine *looking for your favorite cereal in the morning, not finding it anywhere, and only later when you go to do a load of wash, do you find it.*

Imagine *living with your spouse of many years, only to awaken one day and find he has turned into a child.*

Imagine *thinking you are living in a house of cards, or none of this is real, or perhaps it's just a dream and you'll soon awaken, but it's not and you don't.*

Imagine *repeating this scenario over and over again.*

If you are a caregiver to someone suffering from Alzheimer's or any of the Related Dementias, you'll have no trouble imaging this. I invite you to follow along on my journey, with the hope that my words will validate, support, and comfort you.

If you are not a caregiver, my words may seem strange to you, so I invite you to follow along on my journey, with the intent of giving you an insight into the life of a caregiver.

Having been a caregiver, I know firsthand how little time caregivers truly have to themselves. Stolen moments are a very precious and rare commodity. With that in mind, I have written this book in a **"caregiver friendly format."**

Much like the concept of the popular Hop On, Hop Off Tour Bus, **Pick It Up, Put It Down—Hop On, Hop Off,** this book takes you on a tour of Alzheimer's where you can select what is relevant to your journey.

—SUSAN G. MILLER

Dedicated
to All Caregivers

Sooner or later caregiving will touch us all.
No one is exempt.
A family member, loved one, or friend becomes ill
   or disabled and we step in to help, consciously or
   unconsciously, assuming the role of caregiver.

Some do it out of duty; others out of love or guilt,
   or a mixture of both.
Some do it for a short duration; others for what seem
   like an interminable duration.
Some do it with finesse, as if it were a calling; others
   do it by trial and error.
Some do it in silence, not asking for help or unable to;
   others reach out.
Some embrace the situation; others hold back.
Some are guided by religion; others prefer to be their
   own navigator.
 Some find in themselves the willingness to go farther
   into the darkness; others preferring the daylight.
Some call on past experiences; others learn as they go.
Some are aware that if the journey is long and protracted,
   they are at risk of disappearing into the role; others
   remain innocent of this knowledge.
Some do it with a belief in tomorrow; others cannot see

beyond today.

Some do it with their whole being; others with the capacity available to them.

It doesn't matter how a caregiver does it, because all caregivers do the best they can, guided by the knowledge there is not only one way, nor a right or wrong way and, the understanding, "good enough" is good enough.

And, it is not who we are when our journey begins, but who we are at the end, made possible by the lessons learned along the way. Lessons that help us understand that caregiving is about the delicate, paradoxical balance of staying connected, while letting go.

Contents

Prologue

Life has a funny way of happening. You make plans, choose a career, marry and have children. Or stay happily single, or maybe divorce and move on, thinking all along you have control over your life, your future, your destiny. And then, one day, the unexpected happens and your life, as you know it, changes forever and you find yourself on an unplanned journey.

Many years later, you will look back and smile at that incredibly naive person you once were, because now you are wiser and stronger in the ways of the world, and in your own strength to adapt and move forward.

Imagine the shock of having your fifty-five-year-old husband diagnosed with Alzheimer's. That's what happened to me and, without a warning or any experience, I became a caregiver to my husband, then years later a caregiver to both of my aging parents, and then to my mother-in-law, and then for myself, upon my cancer diagnosis.

For more than a decade, I was a hands-on caregiver, a long distance caregiver, a sometimes frazzled maniac, and, ultimately, a competent person who learned how to navigate both the healthcare system and the role of caregiver. Some years after my husband's death, I met a wonderful gentleman and entered into a relationship with him, and a few years later he was diagnosed with Mild Cognitive Impairment (MCI), that would later develop into dementia. I came to call that my "encore."

In the beginning, after the shock of my husband's diagnosis had subsided somewhat, writing became my salvation and something I did just for me—until our neurologist asked me to share my thoughts with an audience he was addressing.

On the evening I spoke, the room grew very quiet, the audience was rapt with attention, an occasional sob could be heard, and I was inundated with questions during the Q&A that followed. But it was the overwhelming gratitude I felt from the attendees after sharing my thoughts and feelings, along with the requests for my then, nonexistent book that encouraged me to continue to chronicle my journey.

> In the beginning, after the shock of my husband's diagnosis had subsided somewhat, writing became my salvation and something I did just for me.

Since much has been written about the medical aspects of caregiving, and less on the impact on the caregiver (as was evident by the nature of the audience's questions), I decided to base my book on my reflections of being a caregiver. It is my intent for caregivers, only recently realized as the second victim, to not be forgotten, overlooked or dismissed. For the sake of simplicity, I chose to divide the caregiving journey into three stages: *Beginning, Middle,* and *Final.*

I suggest readers stick to the current stage they find themselves in, as the next stage will be there waiting when the time comes. Throughout the book, I will reference caring for my husband, my parents, my mother-in-law, and my companion, who all suffered from various forms of dementia. I also will include how I started to prepare for the time in my life when I would no longer be a wife, but a widow.

I have read many books where the issue of caregiving puts the caregiver on a pedestal and is often referred to as a "calling." Subsequently, I have read other books that are imbued with the hint of tragedy and despair. The truth is somewhere in the middle, and I have tried to reflect this by presenting my story in an honest, direct manner.

It gives me great pleasure to share my journey, knowing others' may find comfort, reassurance, find their own unique path because of it. My writing served as an outlet, a guide, a gauge, my salvation, and, ultimately, it helped me stay the course—and to accept being a "good enough" caregiver. It is my hope and intent that by sharing my journey, it will accomplish the same for caregivers who read my book.

or so I thought

Dawn and dusk is the world we live in now;
   not in the brightness of daytime with its promises or
   in the comfort of the evening with its quiet and solitude.

Dawn and dusk is where we will live—made up of
   eerie shadows, subdued lighting, and confinement.
   A world where time has stopped, or so it seems.
   Each day is the same, each day is different; we just
   never know which.
   A strange new world we now inhabit. One day we were
   fine, the next we were not.

This is how our life will proceed from now on,
   OR SO I THOUGHT, but what I came to learn, came to
   see, came to appreciate was:

The moments of joy that living in the moment brought,
   the precious time we still had to be together, the
   appreciation of the totality of our life together, the
   support of doctors, fellow support group members,
   and the gift of family and friends.

These took us out of living in dawn and dusk, and
   returned us to the world; not the one we previously
   knew, but one that we learned to accept, work with,
   and ultimately be all right with.

one

Pre-Beginning and Beginning Stages

CHAPTER 1

Trying to Make Sense of It All

Denial is a normal and integral process, until a "defining moment" occurs and the truth must be faced.

The very nature of the word journey elicits thoughts of preparation— be it a vacation or a life passage—but an unplanned journey denotes little or no preparation, and brings with it an air of uncertainty.

After the shock of my husband's diagnosis wore off, I felt we were both on an unplanned journey that nothing in life had prepared us for. Little did I know at that time that this was just to be the first of many of my caregiving roles.

My main focus as a caregiver was always for my husband, who had been diagnosed with Early-Onset Alzheimer's, but over the following years, both of my elderly parents started to require more assistance, later to be followed by my mother-in-law. Years after my husband's death, I was in a three-year relationship with a widower who eventually would be diagnosed with MCI that later progressed to dementia.

The task of caregiving for a family member or friend with any of the innumerable diseases or conditions out there is daunting, but the task of caring for someone with a chronic, incurable, neurodegenerative disease, such as Alzheimer's or related dementia, is especially daunting. A disease that Nancy Reagan described as "the long good-bye" is characterized by a gradual onset of progressive memory loss and cognitive and functional decline.

One of the hallmarks of the disease is the loneliness and isolation caregivers and families often face, stemming from a lack of public understanding and fear of the disease. Currently it is estimated that one in ten families has a member with Alzheimer's and that does not take into account that only one in four people with the disease get diagnosed. Alzheimer's is one of the most common problems people in their 70s and 80s face.

The toll of caregiving on families is predicted to grow as baby boomers, often involved in the care of elderly parents, themselves move into the age of risk for dementia. By 2060, researchers predict there will be 15 million people suffering with this disease that is one of the most dreaded of all diseases. Some refer to this prediction as a Tsunami.

The months, even years, before a definitive diagnosis of Alzheimer's are often the most difficult and frustrating for family members, who suspect that something is wrong, but can't quite put their finger on what is wrong. It is now realized that it is often a decade or more before symptoms of the disease manifest themselves. It is this very insidiousness that makes the disease so difficult to diagnose and causes family members to question their perceptions and judgment.

Caregivers often categorize this period of time as one of increased frustration, turmoil, and escalated tension. Clinically this stage is known as mild cognitive impairment (MCI), a condition that than exists and can progress into Alzheimer's, when it is then referred to as Early Stage, Mild or Beginning Alzheimer's.

Along the way there are many signposts and clues that something is amiss, but unfortunately the signs are most often only understood in retrospect. Since no one wants to think that the strange behavior that is occurring is Alzheimer's, it is not uncommon for families to chalk it up to stress or old age. Denial is a normal and integral process, until a "defining moment" occurs and the truth must be faced. There is often a great sense of relief that, finally, there is a reason behind the loved one's increasingly strange behavior.

Following the official diagnosis, there is often another short period of denial that allows family members to adjust to the reality of the diagnosis and prepare for the changes ahead. The *Beginning Stage* of Alzheimer's can last anywhere from a few months to a decade. The primary role of the caregiver is that of companion, and life can go on almost as it did before the Alzheimer's diagnosis. Almost, because the person is still present, aware, and able to, with some guidance, carry on and enjoy life. This is the time to put things in order: take trips that you never quite got around to taking; enjoy each other, family, and the grandchildren; research any new clinical trials; and begin the process of adjustment to a new way of being.

This adjustment is not made overnight. Life, as one once knew it, is now irrevocably changed. There is much to learn during *Beginning Stage*, and will set the tone for the following stages. Caregivers need to pay attention to their feelings and intuition, and use them as their guide along their journey and, most importantly, enjoy this time.

Throughout our journey, I never lost track of the importance of how we chose to interpret circumstances we faced. While it often was not easy, I used it as a compass to keep me going in the right direction.

> **Denial is a normal and integral process, until a "defining moment" occurs and the truth must be faced.**

beginning

We sit in the psychologist's office,
   the person my husband has been referred to,
   upon my request to understand his increasingly
   strange behavior that a myriad of doctors can seem
   to find no medical basis for.
   We sit awaiting the results of a recent battery of IQ tests.
   The doctor begins with small talk, inquiring how we
   have been.
   We or at least I am in no mood for small talk.

My husband sits with a vacant look upon his face,
   staring straight ahead.
   "It's not good," the doctor tells us, adding,
   "There has been a significant drop in IQ."
   He wants us to see a neurologist.

In shock and understanding combined, I blurt out,
   "Our life is over."
   And from some place far away, I hear him say in the
   soft, controlled voice so often used by psychologists,
   "Your life is not over."
   My husband continues to stare straight ahead,
   seemingly unaffected by the news.

Weeks later, I am pulled out of a meeting for a phone
   call from the neurologist,
   who kindly shares results after each and every test.
   "It's definite, as definite as it can be," he states, adding
   his condolences.
   But this time I do not blurt out, "Our life is over."
   I simply thank him, hang up the phone, and begin our
   new life.

VOWS

"To have and to hold from this day forward, for better,
for worse, for richer, for poorer, in sickness and in
health, to love and to cherish, till death do us part."

Vows taken long ago, when we were young and full of
dreams.
When they were just words, part of a ceremony.
When the future loomed bright.
When Alzheimer's was referred to as "senile
dementia," and just for the elderly.
When, surely, nothing bad would befall us, and when
love was the answer to all of life's problems.

Now, thirty-eight years later, with a diagnosis of
Alzheimer's, we have become a grim statistic;
some 6.8 million strong.
Our life together fast forwarded and condensed;
both at the same time, giving it a surreal quality.
And the belief that nothing would befall us, shattered
like our dreams, along with the knowledge that love
is not the answer, only a part.
"To have and to hold, from this day forward, for better,
for worse, for richer, for poorer, in sickness and in health,
to love and to cherish, as long as we both shall live."

This is our unplanned journey.

so many questions

I need passports, after all, aren't they required for entry
    and exit from a foreign country?
    What if they ask me how long we're staying?
    What shall I answer?
    And how will I tell them only I am returning?

Or do they already know?
    How long will the journey be?
    What places will it take us to?
    Is there an itinerary to follow or do we simply wing it?
    Have I packed enough or too much?

And what about the language? Does anyone know I
    don't speak the language?
    Who signed me up for this?
    Why did I not have a say?

Overnight I have become a reluctant traveler, not
    wanting to go far from home or venture to new places.
    How did I become the tour guide?

Didn't anyone tell them my role has always been
    passenger?
    Would they even listen?
    Would they even care?

journey

I want to journey to the Orient, ride in a rickshaw,
   kayak down the Baja into Mexico,
   hike the rainforests of Costa Rica,
   take the Orient Express and maybe even Siberian
   Express,
   cruise on the QE2 to London,
   ski the Zermatt,
   bike Provence,
   ride a barge through Holland,
   sit in small cafes in Rome and watch the world go by,
   visit Sedona and get in touch with the mystical,
   travel the United States in an airstream.

So much I wanted to do, so much we planned to do, waiting for this time in our life when it would all be possible.

So much I wanted to do; so much we planned to do, waiting for this time in our life when it would all be possible.
But now our life is defined by familiarity:

   routines to follow,
   pills to be taken,
   schedules to be adhered to,
   increasing dependency the theme,
   mealtimes the highlight of the day,
   bedtime now the shining hour.

I am still young, full of dreams,
   but well aware my time is running out.
   The moment is now,
   but overnight I have been thrust into a world devoid of
   dreams.
   This is not the journey I had planned on.
   This is not the tour I chose.

six weeks

Six weeks from start to diagnosis.
  Six weeks that would forever change our life,
  and our concept of who we are, who we would
  become.
  Six weeks of trying on various diagnoses.
  Settling for syphilis,
  wishing for a brain tumor,
  thinking depression a real bargain,
  imaging all along that it would be something less
  terrible, less invasive,
  not as insidious,
  not so final.
  Six weeks is all it took to take away all our hope.

naive

I thought we were immune from life's injustices.
  How naïve of me, how arrogant of me
  to think that God or Powers That Be would bestow
  upon us special consideration.
  But family genes full of longevity and good health
  gave me no reason to think otherwise.
  Why should our lives not be equally blessed?
  And, if somehow we were denied such blessed fate,
  Alzheimer's was never even a consideration.
  How naïve of me; how arrogant of me.

ordinary couple

We were an ordinary couple once.
Like you, your neighbors, or, perhaps, even your
parents.
An ordinary couple.
Nothing wrong with that.
Married for many years, raised a couple of children,
buried a parent, and lost a friend.
Had our share of disappointments and triumphs.
Moments of anger when we entertained the possibility
of leaving,
but stayed to weave the tapestry of what we were
together ... an ordinary couple.

not ordinary

We sit across from each other at the restaurant,
laughing, sharing an intimacy.
We lie on the beach, enjoying the sun, clearly on
vacation.
We shop for baby clothes, delighting in our purchases,
obviously thrilled to be grandparents.
We look ordinary.
like any other couple enjoying themselves, but we are
not ordinary ... not anymore.

robbed

We have been robbed, as surely as if a thief had made
   his way into our home,
   and confiscated our prized possessions.
   We have been robbed of a relationship, a life, and our
   dreams.
   We have been robbed, but there is no one to report
   the crime to,
   no insurance form to fill out,
   no retribution or condolences to be given.

kaleidoscope

I am looking at our life through a kaleidoscope, or so it
   seems.
   Nothing remains the same.
   Everything in perpetual motion: changing with a twist
   and turn.
   An array of emotions bursts forth in varying sizes and
   patterns.
   Sometimes the brilliance is overwhelming.
   Sometimes the sheer motion is dizzying.
   Nothing remains the same,
   adapting and changing, adapting and changing, as we
   will from this moment on.

known

I have known for a long time ...
   months, perhaps even years.
   Known through dreams,
   known through intuition,
   known the way a woman knows,
   known the way a wife knows that something was
   wrong, terribly wrong.
   But not once did I ever know it was Alzheimer's.

at first

At first it starts out as a whisper ... barely audible.
   Something is wrong or is it simply your imagination?
   But then it becomes more audible, forcing you to pay
   attention, to question its existence, its message.
   Still, life goes on as usual, until the day the whisper
   becomes a cacophony in your life.
   Announcing its unwelcome presence that it has come
   to stay, relentlessly preparing you for the day when the
   whisper will be a steady roar.
   That is the day the whisper can no longer be ignored.
   That is the day when you will know what the whisper
   was trying to tell you.

retrospect

He always dotted every "i", crossed every "t."
   Took his time—thorough to a fault, oblivious to the
   pressing needs around him.
   So when he began to move more slowly,
   increased his level of anxiety,
   I thought nothing of it, barely noticed.
   Only in retrospect.

He was always somewhat messy.
   Unaware of his impact on others,
   leaving a trail of where he had been.
   So when the clutter grew, when the hoarding began,
   I thought nothing of it, barely noticed.
   Only in retrospect.

He was always somewhat unorganized; a caricature
   of the absent-minded professor, critical details left
   forgotten.
   So when he overlooked things, failed to follow through,
   I thought nothing of it, barely noticed.
   Only in retrospect.

He was always somewhat quiet,
   reticent by nature,
   content in his world of solitude.
   So when he began to withdraw,
   become less connected to his surroundings,
   I thought nothing of it, barely noticed.
   Only in retrospect.

standing still

For the longest time, I felt like our life was standing still,
   while the rest of the world moved on without us.
   As if somehow, somewhere, our life had come to a slow
   halt.
   I couldn't define it or explain why,
   but I knew it to be true.
   We had become his parents:
   living a life of reduced options,
   increased isolation,
   safe and secure from the world,
   dependent on each other.

Every time I wanted to invite friends to our vacation
   home, I was met with, "It's so much nicer to be alone."
   Translation: I do better with just you.

He had become his father:
   in your face interruptions,
   no boundaries,
   my time was his time.
   He had become his mother:
   a litany of aches and pains,
   early to bed and late to rise,
   the focus of the day, the next meal.

No longer did he work, nor make any effort to, content
   with the status quo and life.
   And when I came home at night,
   I brought the only world he seemed to need.
   A collection of moments and events finally made
   sense; the feeling our life was standing still, now no
   longer my imagination.

defining moment

Incidents occur, so strange they are dismissed, only to
   be forgotten.
   Or so ordinary they are taken for granted, barely
   noticed.
   Not in any order, but randomly scattered throughout
   the months, even years, before someone really takes
   notice.
   But when someone finally does, suddenly, the incident
   becomes "the defining moment," an epiphany, and
   the ahh!

"How were the signs missed?" we incredulously ask.
   But why might they not be missed when we use the
   continuum of "too young" or "just part of the aging
   process" to assure ourselves nothing is wrong.
   What is it that propels us to this defining moment?
   Our weariness unabated,
   our defenses broken down so that the truth can no
   longer be hidden or denied?

Many moments comprised of collected incidents, but
   always one defining moment—different for each family:
   a car rear-ended,
   the way home forgotten,
   the blank look,
   the question asked for the millionth time.
   And, suddenly we know, as if we are seeing for the first
   time, what we missed all the other times.

decisions

There are so many decisions to be made that it's almost
overwhelming.

disease   Are we sure the diagnosis is correct? What
about a second or third opinion? Do we have the right
doctors doing the right things?

financial Should we sell stocks? Should we invest in
bonds? Is our healthcare plan adequate?

management Should we stay in the house or
downsize? Should he continue to drive? Should we
carry on as if nothing has happened?

family Do we take family vacations versus just the two
of us? Should we move closer to family? What role do
family members play?

friends Should we tell them now or later? Who will
we be able to count on? Will our friendship be able to
weather the fallout?

Many decisions to be made; most clear cut by nature.
It is the *personal decisions* that are most difficult:
Do I leave my job, give up my career to stay home and
take care of him?
An early retirement of sorts?
A no-win situation,
the losses and gains evenly divided,
regrets inherent whatever decision is made.

And what of the *unanswered questions* that loom ahead:
When the time comes, will I take care of him or put
him in a memory care unit or nursing home?
And though advanced directives are in place, will I be
able to carry through with those directives?

So many questions to be asked, so many decisions to
be made.
But the good news is that they don't have to all be
made today.

mirror

Sometimes, I catch a glimpse of myself in the mirror,
    or become aware of my repose,
    and I wonder who I am.
    Surely not the person I used to be;
    she in not reflected back to me.
    Instead, I see a countenance that is old beyond years.
    As if my spirit left one day, unnoticed.

surreal

It all seems so surreal—my husband in diapers someday,
    unable to communicate, him not knowing anyone—the
    progress this disease will take.
    I read about it in the literature, full of well-documented
    cases.
    The doctor speaks briefly of it in his pedantic,
    educational-lecture mode.
    People tell tales of horror, mixed in with comical moments.
    But it doesn't seem real.
    Surely it won't happen to us ... we will be exempt.
    Even as I see this wish for what it is,
    even as I acknowledge my denial,
    I think it will be different.

> **It all seems so surreal—my husband in diapers someday, unable to communicate, him not knowing anyone—the progress this disease will take.**

coming out

How does one tell the world?
>Does one drop a hint over drinks or in between courses?
>Is this like a coming out party of the 1950s
>or is this more like coming out of the closet, or outing as it is known today?

How does one come out?
>Does one simply state, "I have Alzheimer's."
>No excuses given; no explanations needed.
>Or does one give a small educational lecture first?
>And even more importantly, when does one come out?
>In the beginning when it is barely noticeable and easily covered,
>or in the middle stage when signs and behaviors can no longer be explained away?

Different doctors, different opinions,
>each espousing their way as most expedient.
>There is no one answer.
>And, perhaps, it is easier to decide who to come out to, than when.

But one thing is certain—life will never be the same
>after that courageous moment.
>Life will be easier, you'll breathe again, because a weight has been taken off your shoulders.
>Now there is no need to pretend.
>Now there is no need to keep up appearances.

the mind

Look close; no, push it away.
  I am caught in a game of disbelief.
  The mind protects that which is too terrible to absorb.
  Small pieces, fragmented, seem to play hide and seek,
  while the mind pretends this is a dream from which
  I will awake.
  But each morning is the same,
  not even bringing with it a brief respite.

Each morning arrives, like the one before.

alike

We often thought alike.
  While we never finished each other's sentences, we
  usually were in sync.
  Two minds paralleling each other.
  Two minds thinking like one.
  How ironic the day will come when one mind will think
  for two.
  Will I be able to think for him then?
  Understand what he wants,
  what he needs?
  It is reported Alzheimer's patients are very in tune with
  caretakers' emotions.
  Perhaps, we will still be in sync.

talk to me

Talk to me.

Tell me what it is like to have Alzheimer's.

I want to know; I need to know.

But he cannot tell me.

It seems there are no words available to describe it.

It is only when I lose my keys,

forget where I put the bills,

hunt for the millionth time for something trivial,

work myself into a near panic,

reproach myself for my stupidity that he can tell me.

"Now you know," he says,

"now you know."

who is she?

We meet at a cocktail party ... she seems to know me.

"How are the children?" she asks.

Do I know her?

Who is this woman who enquires of my children?

Someone obviously from my past.

I anxiously scan her face searching for recognition but find none.

"The children are fine," I hear myself reply, filling in

details to buy myself some time,

while searching for clues to whom she might be.

Finding none, I ask, "How are yours?" praying

desperately that she has children.

And while she fills me in with all the details about her

children, who it seems I once knew quite well,

I become acutely aware of my husband's plight.

CHAPTER 2

Dealing with Reality and Fallout

It is also a difficult time for the newly diagnosed who has, on some level, an awareness of the disease and what is happening.

It is suddenly as if a dam burst forth and a flood of emotions are released. After the shock is absorbed, there are many emotions to deal with, but families report that the predominant emotion is a combination of sadness and sense of disbelief. Because the disease can render the person him or herself one moment and different the next, it leaves families questioning themselves and the diagnosis.

It is not uncommon for families to get second opinions or to be at odds. Family members often do not come to consensus about the diagnosis, the treatment, or the type of care at the same time. They adjust and relate to the disease in ways indicative of their own style and personality. This often adds to a sense of frustration and stress family members feel when interacting with each other.

It is also a difficult time for the newly diagnosed who has, on some level, an awareness of the disease and what is happening. For the caregiver, it is a time of conflicting emotions: guilt over being short-tempered or irritable during the pre-diagnosis period, sadness and anger about the diagnosis and its increasing responsibilities, disappointment at the way things turned out, jealously toward those more fortunate, fear of the unknown, and doubt about one's abilities to do or to even want to do the job.

It can also be a time of positive emotions: a pulling together and accessing new skills, developing inner strength, learning the difference between expressing emotions, versus acting on them, and, finally, learning a new way of being.

While there are many people who choose not to be a part of a support group, the right group can be a source of renewal and comfort. Although great strides are being made to find a cure, at this time, Alzheimer's disease is incurable. The current treatment plan consists of drugs to slow down the process and possible enrollment in clinical studies. Since there is very little doctors can do, it is not

uncommon for families to have a sense of being aban-
doned. It is a long journey and fellow travelers make the
best companions.

no man's land

This "No Man's Land," in between two worlds, is a
difficult place to reside.
The world we once knew, versus the world that has
become our new reality.
Some days he is himself ... articulate, aware, with the
program;
other days he is a stranger ... withdrawn, closed off,
aloof.
It is this vacillation back and forth I find so confusing.

questions

What is the disease and what is him?
A question not easily answered ... a secret waiting to
be unraveled.
Are his behaviors a result of the disease?
But he had some of them before, now they are just
more pronounced.
Where does he start and where does he end?
When can I be irritated with the same old things that
irritated me, and when must I be forgiving?
How do I draw the line when the demarcation is
blurred, and he just seems to be more of himself?

tired

I am so tired.
 A tiredness that goes beyond, making me wonder if I
 ever will recover.
 How can I be so tired?
 This is just the beginning, even though in truth, it
 began many years before.

It is a collective tiredness,
 made up of increased responsibilities and losses,
 but it is just the beginning.
 I don't want to see beyond today into a tomorrow that
 will be worse.

His dependency grows each day.
 I am gone, replaced by us—living a life for two.
 I am so tired, and it is just the beginning.
 I must figure out a different way of being before this
 tiredness gets the best of me.

first glimmer

Denial ... they will not believe this family of mine, what is
 before their very eyes,
 seeking solace, instead, in what has always been.

I understand their reluctance to see the truth, to deal
 with reality.
 "Dad is fine," they assure me as they congratulate him
 on how well he is doing,
 rejoicing in the fact that the disease is moving slowly.

But moving it is. Am I the only one who knows that?
　Do they think I make these things up or see things that
　are not there?
　"Dad is fine. Listen to him speak of politics, does he
　not remember?" they argue, each one building a case,
　each one buoying the other.

Yet, they refuse to see how simple and uncomplicated
　his life has become,
　focusing instead on all the ways he still is Dad, until we
　play a simple card game,
　and the first glimmer of acknowledgment breaks
　through.

denial

Do not ask me yet again if I have contacted a support
　group.
　I am not ready.
　Why can't you see that?
　Why can't you respect that?
　Why can't you leave me to my own devices?
　I will cope on my own terms, in my own manner, using
　my intuition.
　After all, wasn't it that very same intuition that brought
　us to this diagnosis?
　When I am ready, I will go.
　Until then, let me enjoy these precious days,
　where things are almost normal and I can still pretend.

moments

I complain to the doctor, "He does this and that."

"It's the disease," he replies.

I guess that must make it all right, and I want to scream at him, "That's easy for you to say, you don't have to live with him."

In my rational moments, far and few between these days, I know he is right.

But to see my husband sitting on the couch day after day, contributing nothing while the world goes on around him, makes most of my moments less than rational.

disappointed

He is disappointed.

The children did not ask in detail how he was or what it is like to have this disease at their most recent visit.

I am surprised by this.

I thought him not capable of such feelings, dismissed that part of him as gone for good.

Yet, he tells me there are good days and bad days.

On good days the mind works well, functioning almost as before, but on bad days it is sluggish, slow to recall.

He is well aware; far more than I gave him credit for.

And now it is I who is disappointed for not seeing what I should have seen.

longings

I see an elderly couple.
   No longer am I buoyed up by their bond, or annoyed
   by their slowness, as was so often my response.
   New reactions have taken their place: envy, anger.
   That is what I now feel
   for what they have,
   for what I never will have.
   I assumed, I believed, I bought into the idea of the
   golden years.
   Put off today for a tomorrow that I was promised,
   that I was entitled to, or so I thought.
   I followed the rules, did all the right things
   for a tomorrow that has been reneged.

anger

You get to do whatever you want.
   You get to be not accountable, while I pick up the
   pieces, do the work of two.
   You get to focus on yourself; your privilege bestowed
   upon you by the disease.
   You are accommodated, looked after, taken care of,
   and worried about.
   I am exhausted, alone, weary,
   carrying both of us. Symbiotic victims—one excused,
   one invisible.

watch out world

Watch out world, here I come in my Jeep ranting and
raving.
Out of my way ... I have no time.
Watch out world, here I come pushing my shopping
cart.
Out of my way, I am in a hurry.
Watch out world, here I am standing in line.
Out of my way ... I have no time for your slowness.
Watch out world, here I come, a caregiver, exhausted
and overwhelmed,
wishing I could trade places with you, knowing I can't
and envying you for it.

bargaining

I will go back and take away each and every bad thought
I ever had about him.
Live from this day forward with every irritating habit of
his, without complaining.
I will go back and settle for less and not want more.
I will go back and never complain about his mother
again (or, at least, I will try).
I will go back and be very, very good;
the perfect wife, the wonderful companion.
If only I could go back and do it over.
I would do anything if I could go back to "before."

backward

I thought I was through with it; been there, done that.

But now I've returned to a world I left behind years ago.

I find myself going backward.

To get out of the house, once a simple event, has now become a monumental undertaking.

Something that must be started long before departure; explained, reasons given,

then the wait begins as he moves slower than I ever thought possible.

Until I want to throw up my hands in despair

or simply leave, never to return.

broken

The vacuum cleaner is broken; he ran over the cord and clogged the machine with debris.

The bottle of wine is shattered; he placed it on the ledge, forgetting about the wine rack.

The dishwasher cup is permanently stuck; he did something to it, locking it eternally.

The printer is broken—the second time this month.

What has he done?

God only knows. But one thing is for sure, he knows it's not his fault.

The angry part of me wants to yell, "Hasn't enough been broken in our life, must you add to it?"

The empathetic part of me wants to reassure him, like one would a child, "It doesn't really matter."

The tired part of me wants to put my head down and cry for all that is broken, for yesterday and today, and for all the tomorrows to come.

thoughts

I look at my favorite picture hanging on my office wall—
two beach chairs at the water's edge, catching the
setting sun—purchased to be a symbol of our future.
Now I see two chairs and wonder who will sit in the
other ... another man?

How can I think such thoughts?

dark side

This disease has brought out my dark side, front and
center with no place to hide.
All those years of niceness:
corporate wife,
homeroom mom,
team player at work,
an image I wore comfortably and believed to be true,
gone in one fell swoop.
Replaced now by a new image:
recalcitrant,
self-involved,
and self-pitying.
A whole new side kept under wraps all these years has
suddenly exploded forth with a fury all of its own.
Where has my nice image gone, now that I need it to
support my new role of caregiver?

books

Sometimes it doesn't help me to read the books on
   Alzheimer's.
   It doesn't seem possible this is coming from me,
   the voracious reader, and the one who scours the
   bookstore and Amazon for "just off the press"
   selections.
   The one who already has her own small library
   dedicated solely to the topic.
   The one who copes by gathering all the knowledge
   available.

But, on some level, those books, no matter how
   well-meaning, no matter how inspirational they are
   meant to be, frighten me, leave lingering doubts and
   answers to questions I'm not ready to hear.
   And the people who tell their personal story must be
   saints or darn close,
   not an ordinary person like myself.
   Those people are self-sacrificing,
   altruistic to an extreme, and even when they write of
   their frustrations, their anger, their tears shed,
   it is always noble.
   I don't feel noble.
   I feel vulnerable, frightened, overwhelmed and very
   ordinary.

don't get it

I just don't seem to get it.

I know it's the disease that makes him behave the way
he does, but still I feel anger bubbling up inside of me,
as if he could really be different if only he tried.

Where does this come from, this bit of irrationality?

How much more do I need to know before I can really
accept what is happening?

Should I read more books?

Talk to more doctors?

All moot questions.

I must work on accepting:

accepting that it's the disease, not him;

accepting that he can't change, no matter how much
I wish he could;

accepting that I can't change the course of the disease.

That this is now our life, and I must work with it and
make it the best I can, given the circumstances.

Accepting if I don't work on this, I will waste and spoil
what time we have left.

CHAPTER 3

Realigning Relationships

A support group is where true understanding will come and is often the source of new friendships in a time of dwindling ones.

The impact of Alzheimer's is far reaching and touches the most important aspects of all relationships, down to the most trivial, but it is the loss of the person with the disease that is the most difficult to deal with. Losses are gradual, coming slowly and plateauing, only to be followed by another loss. Families have the difficult task of grieving not just one loss, but many losses over an extended period of time. Part of the difficulty lies in grieving for a person who is still present in our lives—a task defined as anticipatory grieving.

There are some people who cannot deal with Alzheimer's or any incurable disease, and distance themselves from the caregiver and the Alzheimer's patient at a time when their friendship is most needed. On the opposite end of the spectrum, there can be well-meaning friends who offer unsolicited advice.

Friends and family who do not live with the person on a daily basis often, inadvertently, cause the caregiver stress by voicing that the person is "just fine and doing very well." But, the only one who knows the *true status* is the person who is involved on a 24-hour basis.

In the beginning, it is not uncommon for the caregiver to collude with the illness and cover for the person, giving the appearance that all is fine. After a period of time, this behavior is no longer possible or desirable. Pretending and covering up comes with a heavy price.

> The growing awareness of the effects of caregiving has made doctors take notice of the second victim of this disease—the caregiver.

The medical community is in an awkward position since there isn't much it can do. The growing awareness of the effects of caregiving has made doctors take notice of the second victim of this disease— the caregiver. An understanding doctor and, perhaps, a therapist can do much to relieve the caregiver's burden and to help maintain a sense of equilibrium.

The caregiver is caught walking a fine line between expressing the pain and frustration being experienced and not burdening and turning off existing friendships. A support group is where true understanding will come and is often the source of new friendships in a time of dwindling ones. It is imperative to explore and deal with one's emotions versus repressing them. In the long run it does much to ease caregiving. My biggest mistake was waiting too long to join one. I wish I had joined shortly after receiving the diagnosis.

A primary source of one's relationships has been lost and that can bring up old unresolved issues. It is best to be guided by today's reality, as painful and unpleasant as it may be. Two important tasks for the caregiver: 1) find a source of friendship to sustain you through the journey, and 2) at the same time start the process of building a path to tomorrow.

unfinished

We have so much unfinished business lying around—
issues that were put off for tomorrow, never explained,
discussed, or investigated.
It seemed easier at the time.
Life was so hectic, full of deadlines and competing
priorities.
Tomorrow always seemed to be a better time,
promised to be calmer
and surely those issues could wait.
But now the expiration date is up;
our time has run out.
We no longer have the chance to resolve those issues.
Now I must live with our unfinished business, without
any hope for resolution.

become

His mind operates as a child—
    always wanting to stop for a soda,
    longing for an ice cream cone, and
    fast food has become a major delight.
    For Christmas he gave me a T-shirt, button, and fancy
    paper bag, exclaiming, "It's the Grinch, your favorite,"
    while pestering me nonstop to wear it.

Simple pleasures are what interest him now
    and form the network of his days.
    His is an uncomplicated life.
    Early to bed, and early to rise,
    filled in with nonstop eating and other meaningless
    activities.
    TV and movies are too difficult to follow.

A quick nap serves as a reprise for me.
    Politics and long-held opinions he still can espouse,
    but conversations on feelings and dreams are no
    longer an option.
    Friend, confidant, lover and husband—
    roles he is no longer capable of filling.
    A child, a little boy, alternating between petulant and
    sweet, is what he has become.

forgotten

We've always had a ritual ...
    small and silly just between the two of us.
    A kiss as we close the condo door; a private ending to
    a perfect weekend in Vermont.
    Even in times of frenzied hurrying, it was never forgotten.
    Until now ... he forgot, the first time ever.
    I said nothing, waiting to see if he would remember,
    but he did not.
    I told myself he was distracted.
    After all, the roads were bad; the snow was falling.

But deep down, in a place I keep safely guarded, I knew
    we had entered a new phase.
    And all the times since he has not remembered.
    It's as if we never shared those moments.
    I am the only one left to remember them.

regression

His responses are often childish, as is his behavior.
    How strange it is to be a witness to this.
    To see him become, before my eyes, a child without
    eliciting in me the feelings my children did.
    No maternal instinct operating here, although I feel
    tenderness and compassion toward his plight.
    But I also feel irritation and discomfort.
    How do I become a parent to my spouse when incest
    tones play havoc with the mind?

anticipatory

I miss him.

> The way he used to be, the things we did together,
> the dreams once shared.
> I miss him as he sits here right next to me.
> I fear the future that has not yet arrived, when he will
> not know who I am or where he is but will still be
> present, if only in degrees.
> I miss the day he will not be here, and I will have the
> official title of widow, not the unofficial title I have now
> of married widow.

Anticipatory grief is what I am experiencing ...

> part of the grieving process.
> Allowed to occur, the actual process made shorter.
> But somehow it seems a waste of today when each
> minute is so precious.
> Nonetheless, I cannot stop missing him.

annoying

Annoying ... I find him so annoying.

   I never thought it possible for anyone to be so
   annoying.
   Does he have built-in radar that keeps track of my
   every move?
   How can we always be in the same place at the same
   time?
   I can deal with his forgetfulness.
   I can overlook the same question asked over and over
   again, but this ability to track my every move,
   to come up behind me when I least suspect,
   to appear out of nowhere,
   to never give me a minute alone,
   to wait until the moment I was waiting for on the news
   to interrupt with some nonsensical question or piece
   of information,
   to be my shadow morning, noon, and night
   is driving me crazy.

I feel like I could jump out of my skin any minute.

   He is so annoying, but who would understand ... only
   someone who lives with him or someone who has
   been through it.
   The others comment on how well he is doing, how
   good he looks, how lucky we are to still have this
   time together.
   And while that is all true,
   I am a prisoner in my own home.
   I think, some days, I will lose my mind before he
   loses his.

coming or going

I look at family and friends and wonder who will be there
   when this is over? Who will see it through to the end
   and in what capacity?
   I brace myself, ready for people to leave or bow out
   gracefully, wondering how long they will be around,
   how long they will hang on.
   Yet, I know I must be careful not to send out such
   messages or drive people away.

I have become hyper-vigilant,
   not just of my husband, but of the entire world.
   A shared family history of unequal roles weighs upon
   my mind.
   Friends who have come and gone through the years
   cloud my outlook.
   The cast of characters, I think, will remain true to color.
   And then I wonder, am I projecting my fears?

leaving

This disease is taking away my husband, slowly the rate
   inches along.
   This disease is taking away our friends, quickly the rate
   progresses.
   It will be a slow journey for my husband,
   many chances for good-bye.
   With friends it seems there will be no lingering
   good-byes, just abrupt departures.
   I understand.
   But I am still here.
   Only one of us is leaving.
   Why can our friends not see that?

support

I feel so isolated from my friends,
    as if we are living in different worlds, no longer speak-
    ing the same language.
    I sense the connection loosening; the distancing has
    begun.
    I understand and, yet, I don't.
    I would not do it to them—a friend for only the good
    times.
    What are they afraid of?
    It's not catching. Is it simply they don't want to face
    their own mortality?
    That's too easy.

Why should I let them off the hook, to disappear back
    into their safe lives, to leave me, their friend, to stand
    alone, when I would be there for them if the situation
    were reversed?

It's time for a support group, but I'm just not ready yet,
    for that is the step that will make it real and break
    down my last denial.

dwindling

The phone calls have become few
    and far between.
    Old friends, family, and children call less and less.
    Conversations guarded, expediency the goal,
    moratorium on certain subjects,
    cheerfulness the operative of the day,
    duty the driving motive.
    AT&T profits dwindling,
    along with old friends, family, and children.

friend?

I spot her before she spots me. It's my friend I hardly
   hear from anymore.
   There she is in the produce department of the grocery
   store comparing tomatoes.
   My first thought is how does she have such time?
   Should I go say hello?
   But while I was lost in thought, it seems she spotted
   me, and now I see her hiding behind the cabbage
   display.

well meaning

I am so tired of well-meaning friends and family telling
   me how great my husband looks and acts.
   "He seems fine."
   "Look at how healthy he is."
   "His vocabulary is as good as ever."

What is the unspoken message:
   Stop complaining. Stop making more out of it than it is.
   Be happy with what you have?
   I want to shout at them:
   "You see only small pockets of our life.
   You see what you want to see or need to see."

I know they mean well.
   Do I explain the situation as it is?
   Lay out my frustrations and fears?
   My words may fall on deaf ears or alienate them,
   leaving me more alone.
   The longer I struggle with this dilemma, the louder the
   voice I hear ... IT IS TIME FOR A SUPPORT GROUP.

response

Am I depressed?
  Why do these doctors continue to ask me this?
  What response is it that they want to such a foolish question?
  "No, I am not depressed."—A socially expedient response.
  "Yes, I am depressed."—An honest response.

Who would not be depressed?
  Only a person devoid of emotions and not in touch with reality, but, perhaps, that is what it takes to survive.
  But I am not devoid of emotions nor am I out of touch with reality.
  Perhaps, I need to adhere to the standard medical model and buoy up the statistics on depression in caregivers.

I am not depressed as much as I am overwhelmed.
  I can still juggle home and work.
  Why can't doctors forget the clinical jargon and let the caregiver use her own descriptors?
  Why is it that the course of this disease is unique for each patient, but the response of the caregiver must fit a prescribed medical model?

I am so tired of well-meaning friends and family telling me how great my husband looks and acts.

equal opportunity

We are not to judge the patient's behavior,
   no matter how bizarre,
   no matter how obstructive it has become,
   no matter how threatening it seems.

We, the caregivers, are to accept it as part of the
   disease, neither intentional nor personal.
   To understand the driving force behind it,
   to change our reaction to it.
   That's what the books say.
   That's what the experts say.
   That's what those who have gone before me say.

Who am I to argue with collective wisdom and dispute
   well-meaning experts?
   No longer will I judge.
   From this moment on, I will accept and understand
   what I have no control over and work, instead, on
   changing my reactions—not only to him, the patient,
   but for me the caregiver.
   This must be an equal opportunity change.

accommodation

I must make accommodations, the doctor tells me.
   This wise man is guiding me through this nightmare.
   This medical man is partnering with me as I become
   the voice of the patient, the reporter of the status quo.
   This man, compassionate and kind, has not hidden
   behind a medical mask of indifference
   or professionalism, as so often happens.

He assures me I can say anything I want to him but still I
   wonder if it is true ... afraid to test the limits, push the
   envelope.
   My husband is leaving me day by day.
   My friends are slowly disappearing.
   I dare not lose him, too, in an illness where the medical
   profession sends you home to die.

So I agree with him when he says I must not be so honest.
   It serves no purpose for my husband at this point.
   I must learn to accommodate.
   I understand, but when he tells me to make his life
   wonderful, to love and cherish him,
   I want to yell, I want to shout,
   "There are two people in this equation! Why have you
   not noticed?"

micromanagement

I understand what the neurologist is saying now, with
a new clarity.
He says I want to micromanage the disease.
Not in an insulting manner, but as a matter of fact.
Before I might have heard it as a reprimand,
not doing right by the patient,
but now I understand.
This style of mine that has always worked, won't work
with the disease.
I can micromanage from A to Z,
orchestrate our lives,
tie up financial loose ends,
oversee advanced directives,
but I cannot micromanage this disease.
It will follow its own course, micromanaging us along
the way.

hidden

Friends comment on how well I am doing,
on my ability to handle whatever comes my way.
I see admiration in their faces, mixed with compassion
or, perhaps, it is simply relief it's not them.
People tell me I will make it through,
be just fine one day.
Can they tell me when that day will be?
Have they forgotten this journey is about years or are
they just grateful to not be traveling down this road?

The therapist I am seeing throws out a question for me
to ponder: "Do you not think they respect you?"
Is he waiting for an answer or is the question rhetorical?
Is it his way of telling me he respects me or is he just
relieved his patient is holding it together?

Would they all be so full of admiration,
     so sure I'll make it through,
     or so quick to bestow me with their respect,
     if they knew the angry thoughts I keep hidden
     safe within myself?

weekend away

We went away this weekend, the two of us and a good
     friend, and she spent the weekend telling me how great
     he was, how wonderful he looked.

And I wondered all weekend:
     Does she not see that he does not understand the
     dinner bill?
     Does she not see that he can no longer figure out
     a tip?
     Does she not see how confused he became over
     simple matters
     or the increasing errors he made?
     Was she not aware of the constant reassurances he
     needed or the tentativeness of his manner?
     Doe she not question why I drove the entire trip?
     Laced up his snowshoes?
     And spent a good part of the weekend searching for
     misplaced items?

To the public, Alzheimer's is the final stage and the stuff
     in between doesn't fit the stereotype.

the new me

My friends all comment on how patient I am,
>   what a good job I am doing.
>   Strangers, once they know, marvel that I'm still smiling,
>   taking it so well.
>   Acquaintances think it is noble I speak about the dis-
>   ease and share my insights with others.
>   Coworkers congratulate me that I can still do my job.
>   My family thinks I'm handling it all so well.
>   I have obtained a new level of maturity.
>   People look at me with awe and with new respect.
>   I feel like any day I will be canonized or, at least, beati-
>   fied.
>   What they don't see, even though I share it with them,
>   is that I am tired and cranky many a day,
>   and horrible thoughts run through my head.

They seem unwilling to hear me.

Nor do they pick up on my tense body language.
>   Irritating remarks I make fall on deaf ears.
>   It is more comfortable to canonize me,
>   it is more convenient to beatify me,
>   make me something special,
>   almost more than human.
>   For if I were human,
>   instead of this special person they have turned me
>   into, then they too could be caught up in the devasta-
>   tion of this disease.

But is it possible I am too hard on myself?
　Who would not be cranky and tired?
　Who would not have horrible thoughts?
　Who would not be tense?
　Who would not make an occasional irritating remark?
　Why is it I can give everyone else slack but not myself?
　Maybe I am doing a good job given the circumstances.
　Maybe I am handling it as well as can be expected.
　Maybe they are right after all.

why

"You don't want to know."
　"What lies ahead is better left unknown."

Why do they say these things to me—
　the survivors of this ordeal, the ones who have gone
　before me?

Why do they look at me with knowing eyes,
　seeing what I cannot see,
　seeing what I eventually will see?
　What is it they know that I must know?
　What is it they have lived through and will I, too, live
　through?

I want to ask them those questions, but I am frozen in
　fear of what their answers will be.
　So I teeter back and forth on an imaginary seesaw,
　poised to ask, receptive to hear, but settling last
　minute on not asking what needs to be asked.
　Preferring silence,
　hoping downcast eyes will shield me from the truth,
　hide my cowardice, and keep me safe till I am ready.

CHAPTER 4

Redefining Special Times

It is best to acknowledge that things have changed and so has the nature of the celebration.

Loss is never felt as poignantly as it is during the holidays or special days that mark an anniversary or a milestone. The whole world seems to be joyous and the sense of one's pain can seem more acute and isolating. Many caregivers try to hold on to the past and recreate a holiday as it has always been. This places an additional burden on them. It is best to acknowledge that things have changed and so has the nature of the celebration.

This is an opportune time to turn holiday celebrations over to someone else and just take advantage of being a guest. There isn't a caregiver in the world who wouldn't benefit from being a guest. In fact, it may be the best gift family or friends can offer.

Because things are different, doesn't mean that special times can't be enjoyed. One of the lessons of the disease seems to be about the ability to live in the moment. Families have an opportunity to learn and practice this on a daily basis.

memories

Keeper of the holidays and special anniversaries;
   the one in charge of orchestrating events,
   preserving family traditions,
   blending in changing families and new ways.

It's a role not uncommon to women, in which we carry
   most of the responsibility.
   Sometimes begrudgingly, but mostly with love
   and understanding, and joy for with it comes the
   memories, all well worth the sacrifices.
   Memories to be shared in years to come with family
   and those not yet born.
   To validate and honor all that has gone before,
   to soften growing older,
   to hold onto today that is slowly slipping away.

But now I am going to relinquish this role and pass it on
   to the next generation.
   Now I am giving myself and the next generation a gift.
   Now I am going to simply enjoy.

relinquish

There's ice surrounding the Atlanta airport, an infrequent
event, but nothing surprises me anymore.
It seems we're not getting out.
My daughter, tearful on the other end of the cell, well
aware the clock is ticking for her father, has planned
the perfect Christmas to be remembered for years
to come.

My son 2,000 miles away trapped at the San Diego
Airport with delayed and cancelled flights,
my parents, too elderly to drive, but too stubborn to
listen, unreachable on the road somewhere.

In the past, I would rise to the occasion, without even
realizing it, take charge,
check for alternatives,
remain cheerful and optimistic,
careful to keep the family spirit up and
salvage the holiday—a parallel to my role with the
disease.

Only this time it is different.
I am learning I cannot do it all:
shoulder the disappointments,
weather the storm,
keep everyone going.
I am slowly learning to relinquish what I cannot control
or change.

lost him

I lost him in the Atlanta airport ... momentarily, but it
    seemed like a lifetime.
    He said he had to go to the bathroom and I, involved
    in all the details of changing our flights, paid little
    attention.
    But as minutes passed a quiet fear came over me,
    along with the knowledge I did not know what he was
    wearing, and that I should have been more alert, now
    that he is my total responsibility.

This is all new to me, watching over a grown man who is
    my husband, and who once watched over me.
    He returned twenty minutes later, like a young boy,
    sheepish, but relieved.
    We both agreed how confusing the Atlanta Airport
    could be, how much a hassle travel had become.
    Saving face—another chore added to the caregiver's
    job description.

holidays

Holiday time has arrived, but this year is different,
    very different.
    This year we are well aware there's a third party
    celebrating with us.
    I want to grab the proverbial Thanksgiving wishbone
    and wish this were not true.
    Do I hang a stocking for this intruder who has become
    a part of our family?
    Set another place at the Christmas table?
    Ask him to give the New Year's toast?
    Because this I know for sure, this unwelcome intruder
    is now a part of our life.

christmas this year

Christmas this year will be the same, outwardly.
Everyone will be jolly, working hard to please and be
congenial.
Manners up to par, old grievances put aside,
sibling rivalries given the day off,
trying hard to be that Hallmark Christmas family,
if for just one day.
Another perfect Christmas once again the goal
but "perfect" now has a new meaning.

perfect

It is holiday time again ... the season of good cheer,
the time to let bygones be gone,
a time of forgiveness and coming together,
to remember good friends and good times.
A perfect season full of perfect people.

Is that why we've been forgotten,
removed from last year's party list now that we no
longer fit that perfect picture?
We serve as a reminder no one is safe,
no one is immune to life's tragedies.

That there is no forgiveness with this disease is tragic.
That there is no forgiveness with friends is
heartbreaking.
After all, it is only last year we were picture perfect
and on everyone's list.

365 days ago

How different this holiday season is than the last, when
   the possibility of a brain tumor, not too large or too
   malignant, hung over us.
   When a diagnosis of depression would have been a
   welcome event.
   When surely there was nothing really wrong and if
   there were, certainly there was a cure.

Now the world looms uncertain and unwelcoming.
   Now I must learn how to navigate this new world.

wonderful

The Christmas cards are coming in, one by one.
   Everyone's life seems to be wonderful this year:
   new grandchildren, retirements, trips around the world.
   Sometimes, I wonder, are we the only ones whose life
   is not so wonderful?
   What should I write on the cards—
   no new grandchild on the horizon,
   retirement no longer an option,
   trip around the world not on our agenda?
   Life's not so wonderful this year.

black

My Christmas packing for the long awaited visit is
complete: black velvet dress, black pants and top,
black sweater, black knit pants, black long skirt, and
black tights and shoes.
Is this unconscious behavior on my part?
Does it reflect depression?
Am I trying out widowhood?
Or is black simply in season ... the color de rigueur?

talk

They talk, my friends, about the New Year and what it
will bring.
They make plans for a future that, for them, will come.
How can I talk about something so far away when I
don't even know about tomorrow?
How can I be excited about new promises when I have
all I can do to deal with today's realities?
They see their future as bright, full of new beginnings.
I see my future as bleak, full of endings.
Sometimes, I wonder how we can be so far apart.
How our worlds can be so disparate?

unrelenting

I'm filling out my pocket calendar for the New Year.
   Who do I put down in case of emergency?
   This disease so cruel, so unrelenting comes home to
   hit you at every bend in the road.
   And, if that's not enough, when you least expect it.
   There is no respite, no time to forget.
   It won't let you.
   It scatters reminders throughout your life, that it is
   here, it is in control, things are different, never to be
   the same, never to be taken for granted again.

spring

Spring has arrived after a long winter of endless tasks,
   doctor's appointments,
   hopes raised ... hopes dashed,
   bringing with it, as always, the promise of new
   beginnings—
   but not for us.

Endings are all I can see and paramount in my mind are
   the questions no one can seem to answer.
   Is this the last spring the way we are?
   Then suddenly I smile, caught up in the lightness of
   spring ... enjoy today,
   worry about tomorrow when it comes.

**Endings are all I can see
and paramount in my mind
are the questions no one
can seem to answer.**

trip

Four months almost since the day of the dreaded
diagnosis, we depart for a trip to Italy.
Italian landscape passes before my eyes, a mere blur.
Venice is rainy, matching my spirit.
The countryside warm and friendly, beckoning.
But I stay locked in my cocoon of shock.
This long awaited trip was to be a celebration.
Now it is a respite, a chance to gain some equilibrium
before the next onslaught.
Why did we put if off so long?
How were we to know?
What else have we put off for a tomorrow that will
not come?

lesson from venice

I fell in love with Venice.
A city in decay, a parallel not lost on me.
It was magical in a world now devoid of magic.
The rain a slow and steady drizzle,
never ending, matching the progress of the disease.
I fell in love with Venice.
Seeing beyond the decay,
the unrelenting rain
to a magic that remained in spite of all the odds.

CHAPTER 5

Understanding the Impact

It is a role for whom very few are prepared, very few want, and it comes with no job description, vacation, or benefits.

The cost of the financial toll within the U.S. alone has been well-documented over the years. Currently in 2018, Alzheimer's and other related dementias will cost the nation $250 billion. By 2050, these costs could rise as high as $1.1 trillion. The number of Americans living with the disease could rise as high as 16 million.

The real devastation lies in the impact on the caregiver and the families of people suffering from Alzheimer's. There are currently 15.9 million Americans providing unpaid care for people with Alzheimer's of other dementias. These caregivers provided an estimated 18.2 billion hours of care valued at $230 billion. Dollars and cents can be measured, but the emotional and financial cost to families cannot. It is not uncommon, especially among elderly caregivers, for a caregiver to become ill, develop physical issues, have their own health decline, or they themselves die from the stresses of what has been coined "The 36-Hour Day." In the *Final Stage*, I will write about being diagnosed with endometrial cancer.

The caregiver is the one who has been living with the knowledge of the disease, consciously or unconsciously for the longest time. This in itself extracts a high price. As caregivers struggle to make sense, to cope, to hold their head above water, to keep it all together, to take on new responsibilities, it is no wonder that an already taxed system would go on overload. It is a role for whom very few are prepared, very few want, and it comes with no job description, vacation, or benefits. Add to that list, it still is a disease with not enough funding for research, and the majority of the responsibility falls to one person who is the designated caregiver. Is it any wonder caregivers wear out?

During the caregiving process, many factors can complicate matters: previous relationships, unfinished business, old family roles are among a few. It is beneficial to assign family roles and responsibilities based on individual strengths. It is also important to have periodic family meetings face-to-face or via text where updates can be given, a current assessment made, along with ongoing plans.

While it is beneficial to learn as much about the disease as possible in order to understand the dynamics and requisite skills, it is also beneficial to have a clear understanding of one's strengths and limits. For many women who have had years of mothering and or caregiving, there seems to be no respite. It is imperative that caregivers find a way to make time for themselves. Good decisions are never made in an exhausted state, and the world can look much different with a good night's sleep.

Caregiving requires a sharing of responsibility, and it is up to the caregiver to ask for what she or he needs, and not wait for others to figure it out. Becoming clear about one's priorities and paying attention to one's own needs benefit not just the patient, but the caregiver.

specimen

I am tired of being mentally poked and prodded,
    stared at, observed, evaluated.
    My words, my thoughts no longer belong to me.
    Now they have become part of the medical record.
    Does she understand?
    Can she cope?
    How much can she absorb?
    Is she moving through the steps?
    Is she marching to the tune?
    I want to scream, "I am not the patient!"
    But I am the patient; I am the eyes, voice and mind,
    so I, too, must be observed and evaluated.

catastrophize

It is hard not to catastrophize when I go into his
   bathroom and find everything in disarray.
   The bottom of the picture frame lying broken on the
   floor,
   an unflushed toilet covered with spots of dried urine,
   the sink full of toothpaste,
   and the tub with a major ring around it.
   The vacuum cleaner makes a loud humming noise,
   the electric broom no longer works,
   the detergent dispenser is broken in the dishwasher,
   the microwave and coffee pot look like they haven't been
   cleaned in months, yet it was only last weekend I did both.
   The dryer is on borrowed time,
   both cars have passed 100,000 miles,
   various rooms in the house are in dire need of paint,
   the driveway is cracking up with each winter storm.
   It is hard not to catastrophize when I bear the burden
   alone.
   And then I remember, one day at a time, one project
   at a time.

I wish

I am so bone weary tired.
   My mind is overwhelmed and not one more detail
   can it hold.
   My body aches from overwork, without respite.
   A full night's sleep no longer an option.
   My life unencumbered a thing of the past.
   I wish there were someone to take care of me.
   Sometimes I even wish I were the patient, not the
   caregiver.

shadowing

I can put up with a lot.
  Look the other way; be responsible for his life and
  mine.
  But what I cannot do is deal with his shadowing. I am
  never alone.
  He always finds a reason to be in the room I am in,
  to rummage,
  through the drawers, looking for God knows what, to
  check out some inconsequential piece of information.
  And if I take a bath, it is not long before I hear him
  in the closet changing his clothes or in search of the
  elusive something.

A nap on the weekend is an event for two.
  A walk or an errand is something one does not do
  alone.
  He is with me every turn I take.
  My only peace is when he falls asleep watching TV, but
  with the sensitivity of a dog, he awakens if I try to steal
  out of the room.
  My shadow is always with me.

understanding

I understand now why some widows talk so much.

Although I am not a widow in the technical sense, I am a widow of a different kind.

A married widow living with a man, sharing a life, bereft of communication on a deeper level.

Not aware till now of how much I talk in social situations.

More than my share, bordering on domination, not to mention bad manners and boorishness.

The words flow out, uncensored and manic at times.

Wishing to be heard, wishing to be acknowledged.

I go to work each day and converse.

But it is not the same.

I miss the intimacies, the easy conversation, the sharing on a deeper level that comes with a husband.

I am tired of the basics that rule our life and our conversations.

I yearn for real communication, a connection that words supply, a bridge to the soul.

Instead, I must make do with trivialities, fearing the day when even that will be gone.

The time had come for me to pick up the phone, and find a support group.

Although I am not a widow in the technical sense, I am a widow of a different kind.

straighten up

I want to straighten up everything in sight.
  Not just the kitchen in which he has made another colossal mess or his den which looks like a war zone, or the car littered with coffee cups and fast food wrappers.
  I want to straighten up the details of our life that have been left to me as he goes about making these messes, oblivious to it all.
  Finances in a state of disarray,
  wills to be finalized,
  stock options and future plans without direction.

But I am in my own state of chaos every bit as messy as the kitchen, den, and car.

repertoire

There are so many roles I play in this new life of mine,
  I can hardly keep count as I go in and out of them in response to him.
  Some I am well prepared for, others brand new. I have become accustomed to roles I thought I would never play. But the role of warden, the role of bad guy, is the one I like the least.

I find myself locked into a power struggle—
  feeling his pain one moment, understanding how his life is being taken away, but in the next moment clearly seeing he is not capable of doing certain things.
  There is no way to win.
  There are no concessions to be made.
  I am the enemy, a role I have to accept to keep him safe.

promise

Years ago I lay on the surgeon's table,
    breath held tightly in,
    and body motionless as I awaited the pathologist's
    report.
    Would the breast biopsy be malignant or benign?
    The odds were not in my favor.
    I reviewed my life to date:
    one child soon to leave for college; one still in high
    school; sacrifices still to be made. But it was OK.
    I vowed I would find some time just for me.
    The Gods of Fate gave me another chance.
    In gratitude, I promised this would be a lesson
    remembered.
    But life returned to normal, as it has a way of doing,
    and it was a promise soon forgotten.

Years later I lay in the pre-op room waiting for the
    anesthesiologist, wondering if the tumors would be
    benign, knowing either way, I would awake without
    my ovaries.

Once again I reviewed my life:
    It now consisted of an unemployed husband and elderly
    parents with pressing needs that shaped my days.
    Thankfully both children out of college and on their
    own.
    Once again, I made the familiar promise if I were all
    right, I would find some time for me.
    How was I to know what fate had in store for me?

CHAPTER 6

Developing Perspective

I have learned to live in the moment, and stop wasting time wishing it was different.

H ow does one cope?

There is no one answer because it is a highly individual response. The best advice I can give from my own experience is to stay true to one's feelings, go with your intuition, and accept yourself as doing the best job possible. The "good enough" caregiver is a smart caregiver who has learned to balance caregiving and personal needs, and set aside perfection and other people's judgments. And finally, and most important of all, develop perspective.

Simply put, each of us gets to decide how we interpret the circumstance that we face. By the conclusion of *Beginning Stage*, the feeling "this isn't real, this isn't happening" had finally passed to one of acceptance, allowing me to move on and helped me in developing a perspective that would work for me throughout the disease, as well as afterward. It was a journey I never would have chosen, but one in which I learned much about myself, changed my direction, and learned to believe in tomorrow.

Just as the caregiver's coping style is a reflection of the person's uniqueness, so is the patient's adjustment and coping to the disease. Individual differences, idiosyncrasies, and preferences must be taken into account. Being judgmental, bitter, and angry, while understandable, are not helpful coping skills.

It is helpful to remember that each behavior has a meaning and is a form of communication. Familiarize yourself with the following terms: cueing, shadowing, sun downing, distancing, and other Alzheimer's jargon. Be open to new ways of being and learn from those who have gone before you; they are your best teachers and guides. Changes must come from the caregiver, as the patient is not capable of changing his or her behavior.

It is said that no caregiver makes the journey unchanged. I believe this to be true. Already, I have seen changes in myself. I have learned to live in the moment, and stop wasting time wishing it was different. I have learned to accept and work with what life sends me and I truly understand how little control I have. Like all of us, some days I am better at this than other days, but I have made a commitment to change.

Now, I simply ask for the courage and strength needed for the journey, and to not become bitter or cynical along the way. I also hope for a cure; if not now, then for future generations. My thoughts and prayers are with all the families dealing with this devastating disease.

good intentions

I will not be cowed by this disease.
  I will not be overcome or destroyed nor will I partner
  with it in its destruction.
  Good intentions, that's what I have, but are they
  enough to see me through the vicissitudes that lie
  ahead?
  What does it take to ensure one's safety at the
  other end?
  Optimism mixed with reality,
  supportive friends and family,
  unlimited resources,
  strong, unerring faith,
  determination and resilience?
  I wish there were a set formula to follow.
  But like the disease, each person is unique,
  each person left to follow his/her own path.
  But this I know for sure, I will not do it alone ...

I need to join a support group.
  I can see that it is a vital answer to my question.
  The time is now.
  The time was yesterday ... but I waited too long.

whiny

I can hear myself.
There is a whiny quality about me.
Not in my voice but in the way I speak about things.
My spirit is diminished, perhaps parallel to his mind.
There is nothing I can do to stop his downward spiral
but I can and must stop mine.

translation

It is one thing to read about Alzheimer's in literature and
books; it's quite another to experience it first-hand.

He can no longer sequence—a simple task that requires
two steps, now ensures one will remain unfinished.
How many times in the past have I been annoyed with
his failure to follow through?
I couldn't quite believe it; didn't quite get that he
couldn't sequence.
But today I saw it, as if for the first time.
Today I made the translation.

cueing

Cueing ... it's what I've done instinctively all along.

Do you have your wallet?

Did you remember to take your pills?

Have you written down the instructions?

Would you like to go to bed?

Some would call it nagging.

Some would argue that women have done it for years
and men are immune.

But the Alzheimer's literature regards it as the Holy Grail,
almost like a mantra enabling one to get through the day.
What is the big deal I would ask myself, each time I
came across the word, which was very often.
But today I cued in the true sense of the definition—
today I had to remind him to take a bath.

coping

Coping is unique to each individual, almost like a signature.

    I, the caregiver, cope by writing.

    He, the patient, copes by eating.

    Food has become his lifeline, his coping mechanism.

    He is never without it.

    A cup of coffee or drink in his hand,

    the requisite yogurt full of antioxidants to fight off the disease,

    a bowl of ice cream late at night,

    during the day, numerous time-outs for a snack, and in its wake are all the telltale dishes and candy wrappers.

Food, once important, has now become an obsession.

    Two lunches have become commonplace, having forgotten he had the first.

    His appetite grown ravenous.

    Each outing punctuated by fast food stops.

    Each evening's entertainment marked by opening and shutting of the refrigerator door.

    No bedtime complete without the requisite nightcap.

    Food has become his lifeline,

    all he seems to care about,

    all that holds his interest.

    Other aspects of his life now forgotten, but not food;

    it remains his sole pleasure, and his means of coping.

Snatched moments here and there, I write.

    Sometimes during the day, sometimes upon waking in the middle of the night.

    Sometimes furiously with no regard, other times thoughtful and slow.

    I write my thoughts, fears, concerns—nothing goes undocumented these days.

    At first, it simply was a repository, a place to put my feelings.

But now it is so much more.
   A record,
   documentation,
   a lifesaver,
   a chart of my progress,
   my salvation,
   my number one coping skill.
   Now it gives me perspective.

two-faced

I speak with the doctor, setting the tone, asking for
   the truth—no embellishments needed, just the facts,
   imperative that I understand.

How else can I deal?
   I speak with my husband, letting him set the tone.
   Celebrating that there are twenty current drugs in the
   pipeline, agreeing that a cure is just around the corner,
   remarking on how well his self-designated regiment to
   beat the odds is doing.
   What other choices do I have?
   Who am I to take away his hope when it's all he
   has left?
   And soon enough, the disease will take that.

I want to shout

He should not drive but he will not hear of this.
Who has he hit recently?
Has he run over anyone since the diagnosis?
His record remains unblemished.
"For how long?" I want to shout,
but he would not hear, so slowly I take over the majority
of the driving, easing myself into the role of chauffeur.

He wants to continue to do the bills.
After all, he has always done them—
a director of finance in another time and place.
Financial acumen, once his thing, not gone but just
needing more time.
"But what about the mounting errors and the final
notices?" I want to shout.
But what does he care, so I hire an accountant and
become a diplomat when he takes the credit.

He wants to ski, even after the doctor has said it is a risk.
Against all odds he wants to ski, believing himself
immune to the mountains' whims.
After all, he skied for years; what is the purpose of
owning a ski home?
I give up, I want to shout, tired of being the bad guy.
But his mind is made up until I give a performance
worthy of an Oscar, converting him to snowshoeing.

Once I would have called this game playing,
outright manipulation, downright deviousness.
Now I call it coping,
simply getting through the day,
using a survival mechanism.
Shame and guilt no longer a part of my vocabulary or
emotional repertoire as my coping skills increase.

symbiosis

This disease is full of subtle tricks and turns.

One day he is former self and I start to believe it is only
a bad dream from which I have finally awakened.

The next day he clearly is not the man I've known all
these years, and the nightmare has returned.

Slowly and insidiously he moves in and out.

Changes coming so slowly that they are hard to notice,
plateauing until gradually they are accepted as part of
his repertoire.

And the caregiver follows suit in order to survive and
make it through,

adapting and accommodating in rhythm with the disease.

We partner and plateau in sync;

two lives made symbiotic.

shades of gray

I ask him to do something simple, so very basic,
  just to help me out. I cannot do it all.
  But then I wonder why I asked at all.
  Everything is monumental, bordering on
  insurmountable and I feel the anger rise.
  Why can't he do it?
  Why can't he help just once?
  Why must he be this way?

How can I ask these questions for which I already know
  the answer?
  I pride myself on seeing the truth, dealing with reality,
  not seeing denial as a viable option.
  I am learning it is not that simple.
  This disease does not deal in black and white but in-
  stead in shades of gray.
  More than I ever knew existed.
  So I have expanded my life to see and accommodate
  the grays.

This disease does not deal in black and white but instead in shades of gray.

distancing

Distancing ... do we even know we're doing it?

Is there a definition for this phenomenon or is it only
found in clinical textbooks?

I have started to pull away in small measures to protect
myself, not even a conscious gesture on my part till now.

I have become slightly removed, not as vested in the
future.

I see myself less a couple, more alone.

Family talks to me as if he were not there,
not meaning to be unkind.

Once again, unconscious but acutely aware on some
level of the differences, the changes.

He has become diminished in our eyes.

I must watch this; we must watch this.

It is not his fault, and it is we who must do the
compensating.

morning coffee

My morning ritual of a cup of coffee has taken on a new
meaning.

Each morning faithfully, over the years, he has brought
me a cup of coffee.

But now I hold my breath, waiting to hear his footsteps
on the stairs, and if he is late, even only a matter of
minutes,

I fear he has forgotten. I fear he has moved into the
next stage.

But so far, he appears each morning, coffee in hand,
and I give thanks for another day allotted.

So my days have become dependent upon a cup of
coffee, a signal that, for now, things are status quo.

zack

Zack, the beloved family dog, my husband's companion
through it all,
best buddy to share walks and snacks with,
couch potatoes together,
is dying.

Diagnosed before my husband, but companions on the
same journey.
One has amyloids to the brain, the other to the kid-
neys. Zack, the beloved family pet, has amazed all the
doctors, beaten the odds of the time frame given.
And he's taught us to believe in hope,
but most important of all, to not spend the days in
countdown.

few years

It has been a few years now since the diagnosis, much
of which has been lived in shock and frantic activity
revolving around:
obtaining second opinions,
getting finances in order,
telling family and friends,
figuring out a new way of being.
It has been a time of grieving losses, fearing the future,
changing and adapting.
Now on the anniversary of this ominous date, it is time
to slow down and make peace with this disease.
The present needs to be committed to and enjoyed, so
the past can be something to borrow from when the
future arrives.

two worlds

I reside in two worlds.

The outer world that sees me as coping beautifully—efficient, patient, kind, and caring. The inner world where I see me as pushed beyond my limits—angry, tired, annoyed, and resentful.

Two worlds that never spill over into each other. If I try to share my inner world, I am met with:

"It's OK."

"You're just tired."

"Things will get better."

If I try to see myself as others see me, I am met with my belief:

"I am a fraud."

"I am capable of fooling the world."

"I am incapable of seeing what others see."

Somewhere between these two worlds is the real me waiting to be integrated..

fellow journeyers

I see them as we stop in the piazza to a have a drink.
   A couple on vacation...the wife pushing her husband
   in a wheelchair, and
   wonder what the vacation is like for them.
   I see them at the beach club ... a mother alone with
   her mentally challenged son and I wonder: Where is
   the father? How does the mother cope by herself?
   I see them at the mall ... a young couple with their
   children, one of whom has Down's syndrome, and I
   wonder if they ever ask why and how they deal with
   their fate.

I have seen them over the years, but before I dismissed
   them with empathy for their plight, with thanks it was
   not mine.
   Now, I no longer want to dismiss them, but ask instead:

"Are you bitter?"
   "What is your life like?"
   "How does one adjust, make peace?"
   "Do you believe God never gives you more than you
   can handle?"
   "Is it truly a blessing in disguise?"

But I don't ask—it would be presumptuous of me.
   Instead, I watch them, study them for clues, and
   wonder why fate chose them, knowing now we are all
   fellow travelers on an unplanned journey.

congratulations

Congratulations to my husband.

Congratulations to me.

Congratulations to my family ... we have made it
successfully through beginning stage; something
we weren't sure possible in the beginning.

We've made the needed adjustments, learned the
necessary lessons, adapted and survived.

Wasn't always easy, wasn't always hard—much like the
disease itself.

But, here we are years later, moving into middle stage
almost right on schedule.

We know there will be more adjustments, new lessons
to be learned, new adaptions to make, but this time,
we have knowledge and experience to guide us.

And while we are saddened to leave this stage, we
have learned acceptance and become resilient in the
process.

two

Middle Stage

CHAPTER 7

Transitioning to Middle Stage

No one wants to see or is eager to admit to the progression of the disease, but by Middle Stage, denial is no longer an option, nor does it have any real value.

Having successfully completed the *Beginning Stage*, with its task of acceptance and acclimation, it seemed as if we moved right on schedule into the *Middle Stage*, which marked the end of denial and put to rest the idea "we could beat this."

Once again as I transitioned to this reality, I felt like a stranger visiting my own life. I have tried to capture the feelings I experienced as I navigated the issues of *Middle Stage*. In some ways it was like beginning all over again, as I adapted to new behaviors and changing needs, which required a different way of being, reflective of my husband's continued decline. But guided by the lessons learned and changes made in the *Beginning Stage*, I knew we could and would move on and adapt.

Middle Stage demands a lot from caregivers; a lot. It's a time for honest assessment, of continuing to plan for the ongoing future of both parties, and of creating an environment that is conducive to both parties. The tasks of *Middle Stage* involve reaching out and putting various forms of help in place and preparing oneself for upcoming decisions.

This translates into a different set of coping skills, a shift in mindset, a need to develop boundaries defining what I could do, what I was willing to do, and what was simply beyond my endurance, all while continuing to keep my husband safe, healthy, and stimulated. And, it is important for the caregiver to give some thought to preparation for when the role of caregiver ends. As difficult as this seems in a life already overloaded with tasks, it must be started.

There are many services available to caregivers and The Alzheimer's Association or any of the chapters that broke away and went out on their own, has a list of those resources, along with various classes and groups to assist families. Some services to consider are: companion services, senior centers, support groups, daycare facilities, and Alzheimer's classes.

One of the biggest mistakes caregivers consistently make is waiting far too long to do what needs to be done to ease the burden of caregiving. Our neurologist told me at one of our first visits that I had many big decisions to make along the way, and I think *Middle Stage was* the start of those decisions. I began the process by bringing in a companion for my husband. This gave both of us something to look forward to on those days. Next, I joined a support group, something that I wished I had done in the *Beginning Stage.*

The saddest transition for me was the change in my role from companion to caregiver. In many ways I had already lost many of the vestiges of the man who had been my husband, but, nonetheless, a part of him still remained. The change of roles was subtle at first, but increased as he moved further into *Middle Stage,* followed by a shift in my thought process and caregiving skills to match the progression of the illness.

How do you know if the person you are caring for has transitioned from *Beginning Stage* into *Middle Stage*? While much has been written on the subject, clinical behaviors documented, tentative timelines given, suggested score indicators on the mini-mental exam, the best indication is the caregiver's reactive behavior and perception of the situation. No one wants to see or is eager to admit to the progression of the disease, but by *Middle Stage,* denial is no longer an option, nor does it have any real value.

I held onto the *Beginning Stage* as long as I possibly could. I would actually hold my breath and pray while my husband took the mini-mental, as if I had magic powers that would stop the disease in its tracks. My husband also, endearingly, prepped for the exam as if he were back in college. It was only with the heightening awareness of an increase and intensity of his existing behaviors, along with the introduction of some new behaviors on both our parts, that I was finally able to admit to myself that my husband had entered the *Middle Stage*.

> **Middle Stage feels like a holding pattern between Beginning Stage and Final Stage.**

beginning

In the beginning, we did not know what direction to follow.
  Do we participate in a clinical study,
  sign up for controversial gene therapy, change
  medications, move closer to our children?
  There was no itinerary to follow, yet we stumbled
  through, getting off track every now and then, but
  never getting lost.
  I would like to say we sailed through, but that would
  be a lie.

It was difficult. The shock was like nothing I'd ever known
  before, with sleepless nights, monumental disbelief,
  along with fear.
  And just when we were getting used to it, thought
  we had it mastered, come to some sort of peace,
  we entered *Middle Stage*.
  Perhaps we'd made a wrong turn, missed a sign, taken
  a detour?

But we had not ... we were right on time, right on course.
    And all the old emotions returned, just not with such force.

How different it is this new stage with a new road map,
    calling for a different navigational system. *Middle Stage*
    feels like a holding pattern between *Beginning Stage*
    and *Final Stage*.
    Not as good as the past, but not as sad as next to come.

defining moments

There are defining moments in the course of this disease;
    moments that forever alter the course of the journey.
    Different in nature and degree from *Beginning Stage*
    moments, crying out to be heard, refusing to be ignored.

In the *Beginning Stage*, when denial is no longer an
    option, and one knows with certainty
    that something is terribly wrong,
    it is those defining moments that forces us to face what
    was previously too painful to acknowledge,
    and cements the truth forever.

By *Middle Stage*, having grown use to the craziness of
    the disease, it is easy to overlook or miss a defining
    moment.
    Until suddenly, a defining moment, new and different
    finally grabs the attention of the caregiver and screams,
    "I am back in a different shape and form, but back I am,
    so pay attention."
    And the caregiver, in that moment, is yanked from a life
    grown use to, and thrust into *Middle Stage*.
    The defining moment, different for each of us, is what
    propels us to where we need to go for the next step
    of the journey.

fades

Caregiving, in the beginning, is seductive,
shielding one from knowing what's been taken on.
And if the illness is short in duration, improvement
made, the caregiver moves on.
But caregiving for someone with Alzheimer's holds no
such promise.
The most one can hope for is a plateau, and even that
is limited in duration.
Before long, caregiving has taken on a life of its own, as
days fade into months,
and months fade into years.
Past lives barely remembered as the one being cared
for fades, less and less capable.
And the caregiver, picking up the slack, fades from
former self.
Two people lost to one disease.

Letting Go

Letting go is one of my least favorite things to do.
You only have to look in my closet to understand.
By nature, I am deeply sentimental—
attached to people, houses, places visited.
I have never been good at good-byes, preferring to slip
out the door unnoticed.

But now I am faced with letting go, day by day, month
by month, year by year of my husband, our former life,
our hopes and dreams, old resentments, unfinished
business, expectations never met nor can be resolved.
And the by-product of letting go is the space it creates
for change.

Now I must adapt to this man who is my husband, just not the one I married.

Now I must reconstruct my life, which had become comfortable and predictable, to something that will support us now and, me, later on.

Now I must adjust my dreams, at a time when they were just coming true, to something more realistic, more workable.

And I know it is a process, not a linear path to be followed, but instead worked through in one's own time and way.

And now I know, having made it through *Beginning Stage*, I can do this, even during times when I don't think I can.

Still, a part of me wants to close my eyes and hold onto everything I've known and loved.

CHAPTER 8

Indicators of Middle Stage

My life now seemed to be completely taken up with him—a sure indicator Middle Stage had arrived.

One of the best indicators that my husband had entered *Middle Stage* was a greater decline of his functional abilities and a change on my part from fear to frustration and, sometimes, anger. His increased slowness, both physically and verbally, was what alerted me to the change in stages. "You can never hurry an Alzheimer's patient" is somewhat of a tenant of the disease, but living it was something else and gives an entirely new meaning to the word slow.

Grocery shopping became a half-day event, and getting him out of the house was a job in itself. My life now seemed to be completely taken up with him—a sure indicator *Middle Stage had* arrived.

> Until you have taken care of someone with ongoing decline for many years, you will not know how precariously close a caregiver can come to the edge.

The next indicator was frustration. Finally, one day it happened and my frustration got the best of me and I attacked him verbally and with my hand, both indicators of the increased demands of *Middle Stage*. It was a perfectly horrible moment for both of us. While I do not condone such behavior, for the first time, I was able to understand the genesis of this type of behavior, and realize how overwhelmed I had become.

It was in this moment that I knew I needed to join a support group. I was also was grateful I had made the decision to see a therapist on a regular basis. Throughout the course of my caregiving, it was to be the best and most helpful decision I made. Much has been written about having patience and not blaming the person who has the disease. Ninety-nine percent of the time this makes sense and occurs, but it is the one percent where the danger lies.

Until you have taken care of someone with ongoing decline for many years, you will not know how precariously close a caregiver can come to the edge. Later when I discussed the incident of striking out at my husband with my therapist,

I said, "Well, at least he won't remember." To which he replied, "But you will." Truer words were never spoken. It will always remain one of my darkest moments.

Most caregivers are unprepared for the range and intensity of the emotional demands and challenges of caregiving in *Middle Stage*. Caregiving is a continuous process of adjustment to loss and stress. While one can call on many defenses such as denial, anesthetization of feelings and distancing, in the end, the only way through is to grieve the process.

This is accomplished by letting go slowly of the dreams and expectations for a tomorrow that is no longer possible, accepting the sadness, anger, frustration, and loss by finding a way to work through it. The grieving process necessitates acknowledging painful emotions that defy predictability and control, but in doing so, opens caregivers up to new ways of dealing with the situation. There is no timeline for this process and each caregiver moves through it at his/her own pace and time. Having a therapist to talk with and guide me along the way was the best time and money I spent, along with being the best decision I made.

As the tediousness of my days increased, along with the physical demands and mental exhaustion, I finally took the plunge and hired a part-time companion and started to use daycare services. The Alzheimer's Association and your local town government are a good place to start for supplemental services. As I worked at finding resources for my husband,

I was also looking for ways to supplement my income, having given up a lucrative career to take care of him. After much research and unwillingness to give up, I was able to meet both of our needs.

As l look back, I wish I had arranged for outside help sooner. Part of me felt like I could and should do it myself, and if I did, then he really wasn't in *Middle Stage*. Unfortunately for most caregivers, we seem to hold onto the belief that we can do it all, and that even when we do, we haven't quite done enough.

This erroneous belief system can follow us to the end, so it is important to understand it, and remind ourselves we are doing the best job we can at the present moment. The "good enough" caregiver is good enough. By waiting too long to reach out for help, I wasted precious time and caused unnecessary damage to both of us. *Middle Stage* brings new challenges, and it is a time to take care of your health and sanity, so you and your resources are at optimal level.

new role

I have added a new role, one I barely noticed.
　　Sliding into it on automatic pilot, lulled by a holding
　　pattern;
　　his mini-mental score remained the same, unchanged
　　from a year ago.
　　But suddenly it seems I have become the director of
　　his day in much greater detail.

Gone is the simple "To Do" list for the day, replaced by
　　explicit step-by-step directions.
　　Everything must be spelled out, explained over and
　　over again, followed by the same questions repeated
　　numerous times.
　　These new behaviors came slowly, or so it seemed,
　　until one day collectively they registered as overload.
　　I, the caregiver, am the gauge, the internal instrument
　　by which no behavior passes unnoticed.

slipped

He has slipped.

There is more confusion, evidence that he understands less and less.

Favorite activities forgotten, as if they never existed.

He no longer drives much, streets and familiar places erased from his memory.

Nor can he find some rooms or certain objects in the house, even though everything is labeled.

He simply cannot be left alone; a realization I have come to.

He has slipped, but so have I.

My world is made up of exhaustion, defined by tasks and chores, elementary in nature with
no time for my activities or myself.

Running on borrowed time, consumed by the needs of his world, my world is slipping by, right along with my husband.

domino effect

He is losing ground.

Things once familiar are fading to a distant background.

He needs more assistance with the activities of daily living.

But I am losing ground, overwhelmed by increasing responsibilities.

Less time for myself, increasingly accident prone is how I am losing ground.

Like a domino effect, we exist in reaction to each other.

incident

He has lost his wallet with the one credit card in it.

Coming at the most inopportune time with no time
to spare.

My fault for letting him carry a credit card.

"Preserving dignity" has gone too far.

I am frantically on the phone with the credit card
company, while he retrieves my purse so I can match
the numbers.

Minutes pass, mounting one by one.

He has not returned from this simple task.

Putting the credit card company on hold, I go to look
for him, finding him in the kitchen looking lost, with my
purse only two feet away.

"You cannot do even the simplest thing," I shout at him
as my hand hauls off and hits him.

I am frozen in my tracks, shocked by my actions,
startled by what has occurred,

but not as startled as the look on his face.

Years later, when safely ensconced in memory unit,
on one of our daily walks, he hauled off and hit me.
This time it was my face that looked startled.
His gesture did not freeze him in his tracks as mine had.
He simply continued to walk, leaving me to wonder if
he finally settled the score.

next time

I hit him.
  I don't know who was more surprised,
  shock registering on his otherwise blank face,
  horror filling up inside of me.
  I hit him in frustration, out of anger.
  All the reasons why, none valid.
  I am well educated, versed in the complexities of this
  disease,
  and still I hit him.
  I could not control myself, hitting him as my frustration
  grew until it reached a crescendo, and I shouted,
  "Can't you do anything right?"
  What did I expect ... an apology?
  That should come from me, not him.
  I am wrong. I am deeply ashamed.
  But what haunts me, what I fear is,
  will there be a next time?

door

I kicked the door in a moment of rage, leaving a crack in
    the same door my son, at fifteen, put his fist through in
    a moment of frustration.
  I was shocked when he did that,
  wondering where that level of rage came from,
  fearing his anger and the depth of his emotions.
  Now I understand.

props

They lie around the house ... props.

His wallet, devoid of any importance.

Newspapers, partially read but not thrown out.

Stock quotes blasting continually on the finance channel.

Cabinets and drawers lined with labels.

Sometime I want to throw those props out and stop
pretending our life is normal.

But I don't and I can't.

These props support him and *Middle Stage*.

started again

It's started again, those old feelings and thoughts that haunt
me in the middle of night or when I least expect them.
Those devious thoughts that play tricks with my
mind and leave me questioning myself, my abilities.
Those nasty thoughts that make me want to run
and hide.
Thoughts such as: "You'll never make it to the end, this
is too much for anyone, you can't do this, you will lose
your mind. *Middle Stage* is much more difficult, you
will see."

Go away thoughts, you serve no purpose. I shall remember
instead what the neurologist said, pointing to an
imaginary line:
"You are here now, and over here is where you will go.
You can do this.
You will have ups and downs along the way, but, you
are capable, articulate. You will be fine."

So unnecessary thoughts ... go away.
I will be fine.

CHAPTER 9

Dealing with the Impact

I found myself being more direct with family members, instead of wrapping my husband's condition and my emotions in saccharine messages.

As I wrestled with the impact of our transition into *Middle Stage*, the most difficult part was the acceptance and change in my attitude from hopeful to resigned. My goal during *Beginning Stage* was to continue to live as normally as possible and enjoy the time we had together. While the ultimate loss lay ahead, it was as if all the accumulated losses to this point—companionship, a circle of friends to socialize with, ability to travel, a future—were slipping away day by day.

I understood that this would happen, and my role would go from companion to caregiver, and that friends might move on when we reached *Middle Stage*, but, nonetheless, the reality of it all took time to absorb and accept.

During this period, I became a major klutz, tripping over my feet, having minor car accidents, and a few surprise trips to the ER. One person living a life for two is overwhelming. A turning point came for me when I received my second traffic ticket in the same month. It was another defining moment and I knew that I had to start setting better boundaries for myself and address the issues of bringing in help and joining a support group.

My husband was also changing and taking on new behaviors—eating only one food group at a time, sitting only in the back seat of the car, ending up sleeping on the floor in the middle of the night. A good sense of humor and a support group to share things with is very helpful. I had a very special friend, Gloria, and every Sunday night we spoke on the phone to compare notes and always ended up laughing over our "never to be imagined situation."

My husband also had the difficult task of adjusting to his new limitations, such as no longer being able to drive. This in itself is probably the biggest hurdle of *Middle Stage*. Some caregivers simply take the keys away, some let the person do short drives to familiar places, while others spend weeks, even months in fruitless arguments. No matter what you choose, by *Middle Stage*, it must be addressed and put to rest.

In one endearing moment, my husband decided to walk the dog wearing only his favorite lobster boxer shorts. My family was appalled when I told them the story, but I thought his newfound behavior was refreshing after years of corporate correctness. Some of his new behaviors became a benefit to me as he seemed to forget about many things that once were important to him, resulting in a reduction of magazine and newspaper subscriptions to a more workable number.

He no longer cared if I entered his den, and the binders on his shelf, and the contents of his drawers were no longer off limits. Sadly, what I discovered were stacks of clippings from year one that no longer held any value. Also gone was the almost daily trip to Staples for supplies he needed. His den became affectionately known as the "Staples Annex," and it was years before I needed anything from there again.

Middle Stage offered me the opportunity to clean house and get things more organized. I became a fan of the minimalist

> **My husband decided to walk the dog wearing only his favorite lobster boxer shorts.**

approach, and simplified our house, resulting in less confusion and easier retrieval of misplaced items.

It is both painful and liberating to face one's less than generous thoughts and feelings. I found myself being more direct with family members, instead of wrapping my husband's condition and my emotions in saccharine messages. Often I felt in conflict with the dark side of myself. At first, I was repulsed but as I worked on dealing with the unpleasant side of myself versus running from it, I began to appreciate and integrate all aspects of my personality into one.

I was more than happy to say good-bye to the "pleaser/good girl" role I had played all my life. As I learned how to hold the two conflicting parts of myself at this time, I also took on more of a spiritual view to life and the world, which allowed me to stop questioning, go with the flow, and trust the path we were on. This shift was liberating and I began to relax and not fight each day; caregiving became less of a struggle.

The losses that Alzheimer's caregivers feel have been called the "Ambiguous Loss." This is a gradual loss, ambiguous in nature, and it is ongoing until the end. The essence of the person you knew is fading, your life is changing along with all its trappings, and the nature of love is changed. It's a lot to deal with and can make one feel

> **Often I felt in conflict with the dark side of myself.**

lonely and alienated. Finding or constructing a strong inner world is a wonderful way to deal with this.

This inner world offers one a safe haven from the repetitious caregiving tasks and a respite from the job. It is also simultaneously a time to reach out to the outer world and stay connected, if only by email, text, face time, etc. New friends in similar situations are out there and can be a great source of comfort and sustenance. And don't forget about pets. Our dog is a wonderful companion to both of us and brings laughter to the house with his antics. He serves many roles—first as a companion to my husband, then as one to me, and finally as a buffer zone that leaves me feeling a little less smothered.

As losses increased, I started to daydream about my future. I pictured where I might want to live, how I might want to be, what I would like to do. These small bursts of fancy or fantasy, as I like to refer to them, have brought me much relief and offered me small doses of happiness and peace.

What amazes me most is that, even in the midst of all of this, there are still moments of joy and beauty. Perhaps, it is the losses that compel us to look with reverence at the everyday happenings, and see with new eyes. I miss our old life, and would give anything to have it back, with one exception—I would like to bring the new me along.

martha stewart

In the beginning, I wanted to be the "perfect caregiver,"
a Martha Stewart of sorts.
Heaven knows why, I wasn't really a devotee, but
somehow it seemed appropriate
in my new role, and the hidden agenda was ... if I can
become like Martha, I can beat this disease.

In the beginning it seemed possible.
And I often wondered what the fuss was all about:
a few misplaced objects, a lost item here or there,
a mess in the kitchen,
clothes all over the floor—all in a day's work.
That was then, surpassed by now with increasing
confusion, growing dependencies,
mounting responsibilities, and a level of fatigue
I've never known before.

Five plus years from official diagnosis, Martha Stewart
holds no interest,
her name banned from my vocabulary, along with the
concept of perfect.
For now, I know just getting through the day is enough.
My hidden agenda long gone.
I can't beat this disease; I just pray it won't beat me.
And now I know "good enough" is good enough.

.

lost voice

The story is the same, only the storyteller changes.

I've heard it countless times before: from the support
group leader, from fellow caregivers, from an audience
member eager to share her story.

They speak of the tears that flow out of nowhere,
without warning.

Tears greater in magnitude, different than before.

Tears that would not cease until medication was
prescribed, or till someone stepped in and proclaimed,
"We cannot lose two people to this disease."

Something the storyteller knew all along, but was
powerless to articulate.

long hours

The worst time is at night after sleep has run its course
and the long, dark hours loom ahead.

When nothing looks bright and world is full of mon-
sters and one wonders if daylight will ever come.

It is in those hours, while the rest of the world sleeps,
that the caregiver lies awake, feeling alone, worrying
about the present, fearing for the future, knowing that
sleep is a requirement to make it through the day.

But the whirling, churning mind pays no heed,
preferring to stay stuck on red alert.

There is no peace, no respite.

This disease is 24/7.

survivor

Along with forty million Americans, I watched *Survivor*.
   Fascinated, held hostage each week by the television,
   asking myself why?
   Till realizing that in some strange way, unconscious
   till now,
   I related to being on an island, cut off from the real
   world, with the mission being simply to survive.

seasons

We are living in a season of hell.
   The death march moving on, leaving in its wake
   confusion and a shadow of his former self.
   Nothing on the horizon to hold out hope.
   The days have become one like another, begging the
   question, "Is this any way to live?"

We are living in a season of plentitude.
   An upcoming marriage, one grandchild full of life,
   another newly welcomed.
   Bringing with it some relief and a partial answer to the
   question, "Is this any way to live?"
   One season a curse, the other a blessing.
   Reminding me that life is a complex balance of good
   times and bad times.

vacation

I pack his bags, drive us to the airport,
 park the car, lug the bags inside,
 check us in,
 assist him through the metal detector,
 direct him to the boarding line,
 find our seats, strap him in,
 unpack his newspaper, oversee his snack,
 deplane, collect our luggage, find our rental car,
 drive to the hotel,
 check us in, unpack his clothes, arrange his toiletries,
 sit by him on the beach while he sleeps,
 make conversation for two while we eat.

This is my vacation, although it does not feel that way.
 Once there were getaways,
 vacations for two, retreats
 from the world.
 Now we bring our world
 with us.

> ... unaware he is no longer behind me, until I turn around and see him stranded, not knowing which way to turn or what to do next, looking helpless and confused.

brief moment

I skip over the stones, adeptly dodging the incoming tide.
 Caught up in a world of my own, unaware he is no
 longer behind me,
 until I turn around and see him stranded, not knowing
 which way to turn or what to do next, looking helpless
 and confused.
It is painful to witness his deficits magnified, highlighting
 how compromised his world has become.
 For a brief moment I had forgotten the truth that
 guides our life.
 But it is those brief moments that give me respite and
 keep me sane.

option

I stand on the precipice, barely aware of the jagged coral
    underneath my feet.
    Far below the azure waters wait, tranquil in spite of a
    400-foot waterfall cascading downward.
    Straight ahead the lure of freedom calls.
    An option suddenly appears.
    Only a few short steps and the descent begins ... mine
    this time, not his.
    I contemplate for a brief moment how easy it would be.
    Who would know?
    They would assume I slipped or simply misjudged.

sunglasses

The salesman at the Beach Cabana, tall, blonde,
    handsome, the ultimate Maui God, tries to interest me
    in a pair of sunglasses, looking with obvious disdain
    at my grocery store special, as he drones on and on,
    expounding the virtues, according to him, of these
    remarkable sunglasses.
    It seems these glasses are endorsed by the U.S. Ski
    Team, indestructible to the elements, an absolute
    must-have item, plus very fashionable.

Unaware his rhetoric is not reaching me, that there
    is absolutely no connection, he continues his sales
    pitch, which I politely listen to but hardly hear,
    until he mentions the world appears rose-colored.

It is then I perk up and lay my MasterCard down.

frozen solid

Alone on a rock by the edge of the ocean, I sit basking
in the warmth of the sun, so different from the cold
back home.
The sky a remarkable blue, playing off the ocean,
creating ever-changing hues in distinct contrast to
the gray of East Coast winters.
The warmth of the sun, the sound of the waves
crashing lull me into a state of semi-consciousness.
No longer alert, in control—a luxury unknown to me—
I feel myself beginning to thaw out from the long,
continual winter that has become the landscape of
my life.
Still, no matter how intense the heat, how beckoning
the sun, there remains a small, impenetrable part of me
frozen solid.

vacation

The Mexican coastline, where the Aztec Sea meets the
desert, is breathtaking.
The ocean a remarkable blue, playing off the ambient
breezes, the hotel exquisite, the Mariachi music festive,
a friendly wait staff eager to please, create the perfect
ambience.

It is a dream vacation as evidenced by the guests busy
with endless activities or simply lolling around the
pool, putting their other lives aside.

My husband eats in great abundance, sleeps at every
opportunity, and shadows my every move.
We do not have the luxury of putting our life aside;
it follows us wherever we go.

painful truth

We are on vacation.
The villa is lovely, the ocean magnificent, and the atmosphere romantic.
A picture perfect vacation marred only by the truth.
We are in direct contrast to the other guests.
Alone in our house, I have adapted.
Out in the world, I am forced to face a painful truth.
We are no longer who we were, no matter how hard I try, how hard I pretend.

differentiation

I am alone, something I have known for some time.
I am lonely, something I have admitted to myself only recently.
Alone and lonely not the same; a distinction needing to be made.

But first, both must be admitted to.
Why did it take so long to admit to myself I was lonely?
Was I so busy trying to hold it together or was it simply being on vacation, surrounded by other couples that forced me to admit the truth to myself?
I am alone even when I am next to him;
I can live with that.
I am lonely; that is much harder to live with.

just happened

I have stopped writing, but promised myself I would
  carve out a moment here and there,
  but it never came.
  My life is full of his needs with my days planned around
  his schedule.
  And when a quiet moment appears, I am too drained
  to do anything but sit.
  I have lost myself to this disease in my role of caregiving.

Not planned, it just happened, unnoticed as I quietly
  took over more and more of his life,
  and had less and less of my own life.
  Without knowing, I became a prisoner.
  My writing, which was my therapy, simply ceased one
  day, unnoticed.
  My job, which was a part of my identity, given up so I
  could spend the time we had left together.
  My friends, whom I shared much with, no longer held
  the same commonality.
  My world shrunk.

No longer wanting to make conversation for two, or
  cover for him in public so we appear as just another
  couple, or fight the rigors of travel, made my world
  much easier, more manageable.

None of this a conscious decision, it just happened out
  of weariness, exhaustion, depleted resources.
  But now I must find my way out of this narrow
  existence—before it becomes my life.

driving issue

He wants to drive, after all, his record is blemish free. But
that was past, this is now and the disease is moving on.
Selfishly, I am torn between having some time to
myself while he is out and about,
versus being his sole source of transportation.
Thoughts of possible injury to himself or others run
constantly through my head.
We are on borrowed time and time is running out; this
issue needs to be addressed.
I try to no avail; it seems he is fine, end of conversation.

So I alert the "big guns," at our next appointment, and
the neurologist brings up the subject.
Same response I got, but the neurologist does not give
in like I did.
An appointment is set up with Connecticut DMV.
He thinks it is all a waste of time, but coming from the
neurologist, not me,
he goes along with the plan, convinced he will show us all.

driving test

The big day has arrived and he is brimming with
confidence, in between snide remarks
about it being a waste of time.
He will prove both the neurologist and me wrong.
Determined, off he goes with the policeman to show
off his driving skills and prove his point.
Thirty minutes later, he returns full of confidence; it
seems he aced it.
Unfortunately for him, the policeman does not see it
that way.

fallout

The days following the driving test have been difficult;
  that's an understatement.
  He wants a retest because the policeman didn't like him.
  He wants a retest because he was not at his best that day.
  He wants a retest because he will drive no matter what
  anyone says.
  How is he to exist if he can't drive?
  Weeks follow. It seems he will not let it go, till one day
  his car is no longer there.
  Who knows where it went? All we know is it is gone.
  Then, and only then, will he let it drop.

fantasy

He is angry with me.
  He did not get his way.
  I am angry with him, tired of
  always being the one to acquiesce.

> I am angry with him,
> tired of always being
> the one to acquiesce.

  We are locked into a power struggle, simplistic in
  nature, but still a power struggle.
  He plays his trump card, throwing his glasses on the floor.
  I want to step on them, crush them; I can see it clearly
  played out in my mind.

Reality beckons me back, when I realize I would only be
  left to pick up the pieces,
  the one responsible for replacing his glasses.
  So ridiculous is this scenario, that I can actually feel my
  anger begin to drain right out of me.
  He is angry with me.
  He did not get his way.
  I sheepishly walk away—satisfied with my fantasy
  of childish revenge, but promising myself not to get
  hooked next time.

morphed

Rounded the exit, unaware of the black ice, I smashed
into the guardrail, blowing two tires.

Opened the wine bottle and cut my hand, ending up
in the emergency room with stitches.

Spent endless hours looking for items I've misplaced
or thrown away by mistake.

Been treated for high blood pressure, eczema, and stress.

Made numerous simple errors at work.

Forgotten which exit to take off the highway, even
though I travel it each and every day.

Made decisions I've regretted, simply to be free
from them.

Watched helplessly as objects slipped from my hands,
smashing into tiny pieces.

Sent letters out without stamps, paid bills twice or
not at all.

Racked up enough credit card late points, wishing they
were frequent flyer points.

Forgotten to give him his medicine or take mine.

Hit my head on the fireplace, ending up with a
concussion.

He may have the diagnosis, but I carry the symptoms.

the tortoise

"Slow down, you move too fast." Lyrics of an old song
  run through my head,
  reminding me I need to slow down.
  But in a world of cell phones, texting, tweeting, and
  constant communication,
  it is almost impossible.

I know I need to slow down, but he needs to speed up.
  I can survive the same question asked over and over,
  the tediousness of his remarks,
  the simple conversation that comprise our day,
  the shadowing of my every move,
  his inability to do for himself, BUT the slowness of his
  world—a snail's pace at best ... a life at almost standstill—
  is what drives me crazy and propels me to move faster.
  We have become the tortoise and the hare.

meltdowns

Like an alien force or an evil spirit overcoming me,
  one day something simply snapped.
  Meltdowns became my escape, making me feel like I
  was teetering on the brink,
  no longer capable of handling the situation.
  My doctor, becoming increasingly concerned,
  suggested antidepressants,
  but I did not want "happy pills" as we caregivers
  lovingly refer to them.
  I wanted my life back; the one the disease had taken
  away.

A compromise was made and I headed, begrudgingly,
  for the gym, something I had no previous interest in,
  but now it is my haven, my refuge, and where I go to
  exorcise my demons.

meltdown day

He has removed all the items I loaded into the car for
the dump, returning them back to the garage.
He took the directions to the vacuum cleaner, which
took me two hours to put together, and put them in a
safe place, never to be found again.
He has misplaced his watch, on which he cannot tell
time, and wants me to join him in the search—fat
chance.

It is not a good day; my patience is long gone.
But, perhaps the items will miraculously make their
way back to the car, the directions will be where they
should be, and his watch will be on his arm, and all will
be well again.

It's too late, a meltdown is overcoming me, letting loose
with a banshee-like scream.
It feels so good, so freeing.
I wonder if the neighbors can hear.
Who cares, my pride, my dignity are long gone.
I have become just like "Meltdown Maddie," my
two-year-old granddaughter.

context

Today was a bad day. I yelled, lost my temper, had a
major meltdown, said things of which I am ashamed,
but, at the moment, felt justified.
Alone with all the responsibilities this illness brings,
hateful, resentful feelings get stirred up.
I find myself repelled by this person I have become.
I could let myself wallow in despair, and feel even
worse than I presently do, but instead I choose to put
it in perspective ... today was a bad day.

shattered

I watch as one of a pair of our favorite champagne glasses,
solely designated for celebrations,
slips from my hand.
I try to break the fall but to no avail, the glass is on its
own trajectory, just like this disease.
There is nothing I can do, much like the feelings I have
with this disease.
My eyes follow the glass until it hits the floor.
Our favorite set, holding years of collected memories
of special events, shattered,
leaving one glass alone ... just like I am.

fantasy

My fantasy has returned: the one about being rescued
    from this nightmare existence,
    the one about awakening to find it is only a bad dream.
    The problem is I no longer believe in this fantasy, nor
    cling to the hope it will come true.
    Although, at times, I make an exception and indulge
    myself, enjoying the brief respite.

But now with more experience under my belt, I see this
    fantasy for what it is and pay attention.
    It is an indicator, loud and clear, that I am coming close
    to my breaking point.
    Time to consider those "happy pills."

in spite of it all

I am amazed at the beauty of the sunset,
    the laughter we still can share,
    the silliness over something the dog has done,
    the delight we take in the antics of our grandchildren.
    Amazed that in the darkness of this disease, there can
    still be these moments.
    In spite of it all, life still shines through.

companion

He loves him … the companion I have hired to be with
him, making me wonder why it took me so long.
Making me wonder why I thought it would never work.
What is it about caregiving that makes us so reticent
to bring help in, so willing to do it all on our own?
Now two days of my week are freed up, leaving me
time to breathe.
And two days of his week are now a very special time,
labeled "Boys Day" on the calendar.
Off he goes with his new friend, almost like before,
on some new adventure, or simply coffee and lunch.
A happy smile on his face and an even happier smile
on mine.

my two days

Two days of the week I have a new found freedom.
Two day of the week you will find me stretched out on
my mat at Yoga class.
Two days of the week just for me; I feel like a kid in a
candy shop.
Yoga relaxes me, slows me down, focuses me on my
breathing, and readies me for what is to come.
Yoga teaches me compassion—something I had, but
not for myself.

With this new awareness I am more compassionate with
myself, more forgiving of my shortcomings and mistakes,
more accepting of life.
Hiring a caregiver turned out to have benefits for
everyone.

concession

It's taken some time to get used to having a caregiver
in my house.

Something I dreaded, never wanted.

Private by nature, my house is my sanctuary.

Sharing it with someone else, not high on my
priority list.

I held out as long as possible to take this step,
believing in many ways, I could take care of him.

But these days so much of my life is a trade-off, with
concessions to be made, new ways to be adapted to,
where rigidness and holding on don't seem to have
much value or even a place.

So, I took the step, made the concession, and my only
regret is that I didn't do it sooner.

But these days so much of
my life is a trade-off, with
concessions to be made,
new ways to be adapted to,
where rigidness and holding
on don't seem to have much
value or even a place.

CHAPTER 10

Partnering with Healthcare Team

… while dealing with my various healthcare team members over the years, I began to listen and rely on my own voice, having profited from their collective wisdom.

Whenever I have a speaking engagement, during the Q&A period invariably the topic turns to the subject of healthcare professionals. By the very nature of the disease, relationships that caregivers have with healthcare professionals are complex and long in duration. Add into that equation that both parties have their own concerns and agenda, it is no wonder visits can become strained at times. I wonder, sometimes, if the medical profession can feel this discomfort, as it seems to me most of what does not fall under the realm of clinical can be met with a certain level of resistance.

The very fact that today's doctors are working under strict time guidelines allows less time for the non-medical aspects and concerns that go along with the diagnosis. Dancing as fast as they can in this medical model driven by insurance companies, I am sure patients are missing the comfort of the old days, perhaps even the doctors, too.

Naively, at first, I expected our neurologist to be all things to us, often causing tension in both of us. In the Beginning Stage there was much to learn, absorb, accept, and do, and the support of healthcare professionals is critical. My disappointment in the lack of time available during visits led to feelings of disappointment, and occasionally abandonment. Interestingly enough, those feelings parallel my feelings about the disease.

Middle Stage seems, to me, more of a holding pattern, and one in which the neurologist has less of a role. At this point, I realized the necessity of building a supplemental healthcare team to support us. Nonetheless, I will always be grateful for his support and especially on one of our first visits when he took me aside and drew an imaginary line with two points. He showed me where I was and where I was going, and told me I was bright, articulate, and direct. I would be fine. Throughout my journey, I repeated his words like a mantra. He also prepared me early on for the upcoming tough decisions I would have to make.

Our visits to our primary physician, who had known us for a long time, were more focused on the emotional aspects of the disease. His kindness and support were welcomed, and he was a vital of our medical team.

My psychologist became my lifeline, and my source for developing coping skills, and maintaining a healthy perspective, along with being a wonderful source of comfort. It was reassuring to me to know I would not be alone on this journey and that I was free to voice any feelings without judgment. It was here that I learned to face my fears, ugly thoughts, and raw emotions, construct boundaries, gain the strength to put aside other's opinions and listen to my own, and begin the process of developing a new life for me in the future, while simultaneously dealing with what life had dealt me.

Without his help and support, I would not have made it through in the good shape that I did. I am forever thankful for the decision to seek counseling for myself and for the time we spent together.

I also sought out an Alzheimer's psychologist specialist, who I referred to as the "Alzheimer's Guru." In his office, I was able to learn about and understand the intricacies of the disease, which enabled me to better understand and deal with my husband's behavior. Best of all, I never had to go to great lengths for him to get the picture. Most amazing was his uncanny sense of timing. During one visit, he wanted me to explore the issue of wandering, to which I assured him this was not an issue. The very next week I lost my husband, for what seemed like an eternity, in Grand Central Station.

My support group leader became a weekly lifesaver. Her unwavering support, compassion, group skills, and commitment made all the difference. I was slow to join a group, but quickly learned its value. A support group is a necessity, but the problem lies in finding the correct one.

Do not give up the first or even second time around because, eventually, you will find the perfect fit for you. The real value of the group, aside from the friendships formed with those in the same situation, lies in the free, non-judgmental expressions of your feelings, and the ability to learn from those who have gone before you, commiserate with those who are in the place you are in, and welcome the new members and, by doing so, see the progress you have made. It also offers caregivers an opportunity to watch as others struggle with issues, which are not presently theirs, offering good preparation for the future.

Many of the women in the group became personal friends. After all, who knows better than one who is going through the same thing?

Support groups are a safe haven, where you can talk about all your feelings without fear of judgment or being told, "You shouldn't feel that way. After all, your spouse has Alzheimer's and can't help it." This may all be true, but it serves no helpful purpose. I am always amazed at what is laid out on the table during these meetings, with never an eyebrow raised or critical comment made. This is the best support a caregiver can receive. Whether you physically join a group or go online, the benefits are lifesaving.

My healthcare team included a private caregiver I hired to take my husband on outings two days a week. This offered him male companionship, interesting trips, and a chance to get away from the house and me. It turned out to be one of the best investments I've ever made and was beneficial for both of us. I don't know who looked forward to those days more. Another useful supplement was to take him to the Senior Center every now and then for a change of pace.

Later on, the staff of the Memory Care Unit, in the assisted living facility I placed my husband in, became a part of the team. Their experience and expertise was most helpful during the final months, and Hospice was a source of strength and guidance for me as we faced the end together.

When dealing with the various healthcare professionals who made up our team, I have tried very hard to be respectful of their time by coming with a list of concerns, outline of my husband's current state, and the knowledge that we are just one of many patients. *Beginning Stage* is a flurry of diagnosis and treatment plan options, but during *Middle Stage* there is a shift to developing new strategies and attending to increased symptoms and behaviors. Documented research on caregiver burden shows an increase during *Middle Stage.*

Caregivers have wider concerns, while physicians are focused on treatment. Taking care of someone with Alzheimer's needs to be a partnership that covers both the person with Alzheimer's and the caregiver, making it imperative to build a team to cover all the bases.

No matter what my feelings are on any given day, I am forever grateful and indebted to my healthcare team. After all, it is they who convinced me to bring in a day companion for my husband and on alternate days, enroll him in an Alzheimer's daycare program, join a support group, and consider and finally take antidepressants, and place him in respite care for two weeks. An interesting outcome of all of this was, while dealing with my various healthcare team members over the years, I began to listen and rely on my own voice, having profited from their collective wisdom.

disconnect

Disconnect:
when the synapses are covered with amyloids,
rendering them nonfunctioning,
when families cannot make the distinction between
strange behavior and the disease,
when the one afflicted is incapable of change, thinking
they are just fine,
when caregiver's emotions overcome the rational mind,
when the helping profession has run out of options.

my therapist, my luxury

I sit in my therapist's office, far away from the demands
of the disease,
but the concerns sit there right next to me, following
me wherever I go.
His office is different—time slows down, I slow down.
The atmosphere is tranquil, no matter what is being
discussed, a safe haven of sorts.
Eventually I follow suit and become tranquil.
The agenda belongs to me; the focus is on me.
I have the luxury of discussing my needs, not my
husband's.
This time belongs just to me.

In reality this "luxury" is really a "necessity" in order for
me to navigate the disease and stay sane.
BUT, the insurance company does not always see it
that way.
Perhaps I shall drop my husband off at the insurance
company for a day's stay; by the very next day, coverage
will not be an issue and a new DSM* will be in place.

*Diagnostic Statistical Manual where codes are described to be used
for billing purposes. There are specific codes that relate to Alzheimer's
reimbursement.

best interest

Sitting in my therapist's office, unhappy with him for
   what I perceive as a minor offense,
      unhappy with myself for my response to him,
      we try to iron it out, uncover issues, but to no avail.
      "It's in your best interest," he explains.
      I leave feeling hurt and for days his words toss around in
      my head; words and concepts that are unfamiliar to me.
      And why wouldn't they be, used to putting other
      people's needs first, never occurring that I could have a
      best interest?
      And if I had a best interest, certainly this disease has
      nullified it, leaving me without choices.

Choices exist even when we cannot see them, feel them,
   or be aware of their existence.
      Perhaps, going forward, I should take my therapist's
      comment and consider what is in my best interest;
      a point he has been driving home over the past few
      months—unsuccessful till now.

who's the stupid one here?

"He's stupid." That's what I tell the therapist in a moment
   of exhaustion.
      Tired, worn out, and fed up with my husband's
      ongoing behavior:
      never finding the correct car door, winding up in
      the back seat or cargo area or, worse yet,
      following right behind me to the driver's door,
      standing there with the now infamous blank stare,
      asking the same questions over and over, telling the
      same story, the only story.

"He's not stupid; he has Alzheimer's." This is his reply,
given in a nonjudgmental tone.
But I forgot ... as if it was something one could forget,
but forget I did.
In my exhaustion and annoyance, I reacted as if my
husband was stupid.
Thank goodness I have my
therapist to remind me, to
keep me on track.

> **In my exhaustion and annoyance, I reacted as if my husband was stupid.**

speaks

She speaks to me with softness in her voice,
this young psychologist I have been referred to
regarding research on caregivers.
I feel an instant connection—visceral in nature, coming
through the phone.

She is someone who goes beyond the research data.
We talk of adaptive styles,
the influence of genetics versus learned behavior.
She says it's a different kind of loss.
Nothing I haven't heard already, but from her I hear it
differently.

She comments on how difficult it must be, and I agree,
with short stories to punctuate the point.
I am careful not to burden her.

She is not the first to reach out in kindness, but she is the
first to evoke tears.
Thank God for the privacy of the phone. This woman
has made a small hole in my protective armor and in
my need to hold it all together.

lunar moon

I sit in the office of the psychiatrist, the one who will
  do periodic medication checks, now that I have wisely
  acquiesced and started on medication.
  He wants to know my background, so I tell him our
  story, connecting past and present;
  something I have become quite adept at.

He listens intently, while I wonder if he is really interested
  or it is just his job.
  Quickly, I catch myself. Does it really matter?
  Nonetheless, I try to be succinct, highlighting only the
  important, not wanting to sound whiny or martyr-like.
  I tell him I am afraid of my anger and the potential
  damage it could do.

"Who sustains you?" he asks.
  So overwhelmed by the question, my mind cannot go
  on a search for an answer.
  Sustain me—it has been too long to even remember
  what that is, and as if he could read my thoughts, he
  paints a picture with words of where I reside:
  a lunar landscape, barren with only craters that I am in
  danger of falling into if I am not observant.
  There is not enough oxygen to sustain me, nor is there
  an anchor. I am adrift.

I feel the sensation of not being connected, of floating.
  Slowly he brings me back to reality, but I am not ready.
  I want to linger in this place that feels so familiar,
  finding myself both fascinated and repelled—parallel to
  my feelings about the disease.

guru

I am seeing an Alzheimer's guru. At least that's how
my friend billed him.
Wise, older, philosophical, and experienced with the
disease,
he has the perfect credentials.
But I am skeptical; I know the drill too well by now.
He will tell me the usual:
Coping tips to make life easier, advise me to feel the pain,
deal with my anger, and then he will monitor my
answers to his list of questions,
the final one being asking me to rate the present
quality of my life.
The inaneness of that final question nearly pushing me
beyond my limits.

When he is done, I will tell him what I told the others:
"You can teach me all the coping skills available, help
me understand and develop strategies,
but you cannot bring my husband back."

To my surprise, he does not offer coping skills, suggest
support groups,
nor fault me for not fully having come to terms with
my situation.
What he does, front and center, is outline what is coming,
advise me to put a Safe Return bracelet on my husband,
place him on a list for future assisted living,
begin to get my new life in order,
and shift the focus back onto me.

neurologist

Today I went to see our neurologist, who I am grateful to
have, to talk about the future.
But he was reluctant, after all, he cannot predict the
future and Alzheimer's is not a disease of precise
timetables.
I sensed his reluctance, but now we are in *Middle Stage*
and things are different.

Changing tack, I told him I had a therapist for the
emotional issues,
and what I needed from him was someone to tell me
the truth about tomorrow.
I told him I knew he didn't have all the answers,
but I was not content to make do,
nor was I bailing out, but that life with my husband had
become increasingly frustrating.
I needed some kind of a timeline.

He listened politely, then kindly reprimanded me for
making myself upset.
What purpose did it serve?

Then I told him what I had known all along, but had been
too polite to articulate until now.
The trouble with doctors in white coats is no matter
how many patients they deal with during the day, at
night they get to go home, leaving Alzheimer's behind.

another expert

We have seen another expert on the opposite coast,
    a world renounced expert on cutting edge procedures,
    to find out if my he is a candidate, to assess the risks,
    to learn the details.
    The conversation eventually turns to care and he
    assures me, like our neurologist at home,
    the best place for care is at home.
    I silently wonder, have these doctors ever taken care
    of anyone at home, or do they simply dispense advice
    from the safety of their offices?
    It seems they know nothing about the exhaustion of
    having one's home turned into a hospital, or what it's
    like to live 24/7 with someone who is not present.

What is best for the patient, may not be best for the
    caregiver.
    I have seen, firsthand, the devastation to families,
    witnessed the exhaustion, the tears that will not
    stop, and the feeling that one cannot go on one
    more moment.
    How many lives must be sacrificed to this disease
    before the doctors in white coats get it?
    I respect their medical acumen,
    know their intentions are well meant, but medical
    degrees and intentions aside,
    until you've lived it, you just don't get it!

> **It seems they know nothing about the exhaustion of having one's home turned into a hospital, or what it's like to live 24/7 with someone who is not present.**

imagination

Is it my imagination or is it real?

I sense our neurologist backing off, eager to turn us
over to the nurse practitioner.

After all, it is managed care efficient, and my husband
has transitioned into the No Man's Land of *Middle Stage.*

I am aware of new losses, mounting spatial difficulties,
growing confusion, increased deficits.

I sense our neurologist does not want to talk about
it. He is briefer, to the point. If the current medication
does not work, try another.

End of discussion.

The tone of the visit has subtly changed to less
hopeful, less guidance, increasing silence.

I wonder if this is how it will be going forward.

Is this how doctors protect themselves from the
inevitable, when their healing powers no longer serve
them?

Is distancing their coping mechanism of choice?

I cannot blame them.

After all, how long can one tolerate being in a situation
almost devoid of resources?

But I am still here, the other half of the patient, and I
need him to stay present, to enlarge his comfort zone,
and to treat this disease in its entirety.

zen

We speak, the neurologist and I, during one of our updates.
    I tell him I often react to my husband as if he didn't
    have Alzheimer's.
    I am well aware of what this is—my own form of denial.
    I am aware of old defenses that no longer serve me,
    but remain in place.

I am stuck; I have plateaued.
    He tells me I need to go more with the flow as these
    stages change, as losses increase.
    He speaks of Zen and the Buddhist approach to loss.
    Going straight to transcendence is more of what I had
    in mind.
    I resist the pain, the sadness, well aware this is what
    keeps me blocked,
    and keeps me from going with the flow.

changing

Am I the one changing or is it the neurologist in response
    to me?
    Does he finally sense my exhaustion is more emotional
    than physical?
    The wearing down of my resources, depleted by the
    monotony of my days,
    by the feeling of my husband being imprisoned in
    Middle Stage,
    and myself in the collective confinement and shrinking
    of our existence?

This visit has taken a turn, a new direction.
    He is alternately concerned and brusque,
    wavering back and forth between the needs of my
    husband and me.

charts

She comes, Nurse Ratchet in disguise, to aid me in my
   attempt to deal with this disease—
   specifically the non-medical aspects, upon request
   from our neurologist, who, it seems, only wishes to
   deal with the medical aspects.
   She does not listen to what I say; she has her own agenda.
   Instead, she pulls out her charts, admonishes me for
   things I still let him do,
   so sure he is headed for next stage.
   After all, it's all there in her charts.

Yes, it will progress, I am well aware, but right now,
   it has not.
   She changes tack and asks about daycare, what are
   my plans, right after I tell her
   about all the activities I've arranged to give meaning
   to his day.
   She will not listen; she sees only what's in her charts.
   And I will not turn my husband's dignity over to her
   and her charts.

advice

"Just take him home and love him." That's how I know
   my visit with the neurologist
   is coming to the end.
   It is his sage advice dispensed at the close of each visit.
   But what is the translation, what does it mean?
   There is no hope, there is nothing more I can do?
   And how does it apply to me?
   Am I simply to be a courtesan or just the devoted wife?
   Does it imply I am not seeing the big picture, grasping
   the situation in its entirety?
   Or is it simply reality wrapped up in nice words?

message

I did not understand the comment from our neurologist,
"Just take him home and love him."
I silently admonished him for being insensitive,
chauvinistic, not in touch with the reality of our
situation, or worse yet, medically wiping his hands
of our situation.
Now further along into *Middle Stage,* I hear the
message differently, and understand the context in
which it was given.
His hope, is at the end, I have no regrets.
And now, with the clarity that time affords, I see the
kindness behind it,
not just for my husband, but for me, the caregiver.

truth

It has taken a long while to see the light, to understand
the growing indifference of
the neurologist now that we are in *Middle Stage*.
In Beginning Stage, we were a team, a partnership,
going through the diagnosis step by step.
Then the focus became educational, to bring the
caregiver up-to-date,
followed by medication checks.

Now firmly planted in *Middle Stage,* the visits are
few and far between.
No follow-up cards arrive in the mail.
Maintenance is all we can hope for, and even that is
wishful.
I don't feel like part of a team anymore ... more like an
annoyance, whisked in and out.
In part, dictated by insurance factors, along with
acceptance of the truth;
nothing more can be done.
We were dead-on with diagnosis.
Why did it take me so long to see?

he's gone

"He's gone." That is what the neurologist said to me
on our last visit.
He's gone.
I find myself referring to him in my mind as "that man."
After all, he is no longer the man I married.
He's become "that man."
I tell the doctor he still presents well, to which he replies,
"A pianist can still play, even if it's only one tune."

Our son, on a recent visit home exclaims, "Dad is just
  a shell of himself."
  And I am careful not to add, a shattered shell.
  He's gone ... a unanimous decision on all our parts.
  But where has he gone?

understanding

His neurologist cannot save him, nor can I,
  an understanding I have come to
  midway into the disease.
  Making for a different kind of relationship—no longer
  asking about medical
  advances or clinical trials, allowing me now to hear
  in a new way,
  making space for words spoken and unspoken.

Objectives have shifted.
  Hope has been replaced by a deep sense of sadness,
  a grieving for what might have been possible.
  Helping me to finally accept the diagnosis in its
  entirety, and for preparation for the inevitable.
  My husband is leaving me.
  Will our neurologist be next, now that the bulk of his
  work is done?

> **Hope has been replaced by a deep sense of sadness, a grieving for what might have been possible.**

surprised

Surprised, that's what I am, by this most recent visit to
the neurologist.

The focus was not on my husband.

No helpful hints, suggestions offered.

Not even once mentioning the parting line—"Keep him
home as long as you can."

Instead, the focus was on me.

It seems I need to start to prepare myself for the
difficult decisions coming up, think about my life going
forward, understand my limitations, and connect with
my intuition.

For the first time, I felt like a person, not just a caregiver.

dilemma

"He needs a colonoscopy; it's that time again."

That is what our internist recommends at each and
every visit.

I have stated my position: I see no reason why I would
put my husband through this,

along with the horrors of prep and procedure.

And, if the news were bad, why with his condition,
would I subject him to more,

much less the risk of anesthesia?

He listens, taking it all in, seeming to understand, but
on the very next visit, he starts in again.

To him, I must seem noncompliant, the very worst
thing a patient can be,

not to mention, cold and uncaring.

I wish he could come to my support group where this
   topic and similar others
   have been hashed around innumerable times.
   Surrounded by caregivers in the same situation has
   helped prepare me for this decision,
   and given me the insight and fortitude to take this
   stand.

Years of being a good patient, years of being blessed
   with this special man as our doctor, our relationship
   is at risk of being eroded, by conflicting options.
   Medicine is about saving lives, but what about quality
   of life?
   I cannot in good faith risk my husband accelerating
   faster, trading off time still available,
   nor do I wish to jeopardize a relationship that up to
   this point has been positive.
   On the next visit, he lets me know he has given it more
   thought, and concurs and supports my decision, adding
   he has learned something new along the way.

experts

I want to run to the "experts," whoever they may be,
   wherever they may be, and ask,
   "What is it I should do?" and a million other questions
   that swirl about in my mind.
   But, one thing I have found to be true, one thing I have
   come to understand:
   The experts are not found just in white coats or
   therapeutic rooms, or over kitchen tables
   with friends or family, or even in support groups.
   The expert is in each and every one of us, just waiting
   to be heard.

rehearsal

Our internist of twenty years is leaving,
   a retirement of sorts, a sabbatical, I secretly hope.
   Burned out by the demands of managed care and less
   time for patients, it is time for a change.
   Perhaps he needs to do things not yet done.
   It doesn't matter the reason why ... bottom line, he is
   leaving.

He has always been there; a unique, gifted doctor
   possessed of abundant sensitivity,
   caring and goodwill.
   A doctor who upon my husband's diagnosis became
   my safety net,
   someone who
   would oversee care for me if I became sick—
   a caregiver's biggest fear.
   He is leaving, just like my husband.
   I feel a sense of sadness and longing for what was,
   tinged with feelings of abandonment;
   the same feelings I have about my husband.

He is leaving and I shall compare all future doctors to
   him, never letting one get close again.
   He tells me I will be fine. But will I?
   The rational answer is yes, and I know that.
   The non-rational part of me thinks surely this is
   another dream from which I will awaken.
   But it is not a dream, nor is my husband's condition
   a dream.
   Now I have to say good-bye to two people so dear to me.
   This feels like a rehearsal.

peace

Somewhere, somehow, I must make peace with my
impatience and unrealistic
expectations of the medical profession.
They cannot always be the bad guys, the villains.
After all, we are partners working in allegiance.

I am not of the generation that put blind faith in its doctors,
never spoke up, never questioned.
Nonetheless, I know my persistence for answers, when
there are none,
in a world of managed care that leaves no time for
questions, much less answers
is a source of irritation.

There needs to be a new medical model for handling this
disease, with time built into the visit for caregiver's
needs and concerns.

learning

I am learning ... ever so slowly ... but learning I am.
Going with the flow, accepting, letting go is making my
days easier.
I cannot control this disease; I cannot control the future.
So much is out of my hands, out of my control.

Why did it take me so long to realize this?
Then I laugh and in my newfound wisdom say to myself,
"Don't be so judgmental. You are doing the best you can."
I can see tomorrow without such fear.
I can appreciate today for what it brings.
I can trust that it will all play out and I will be okay.
I am learning.

CHAPTER 11

Drawing Comfort from Our Relationships

New friends will be the friends who GET IT, who support you, and make you not feel so alone.

The family unit is an interesting dynamic; throw in caregiving, and it can become even more interesting. Based on my own family and the stories I have heard from numerous caregivers, it seems once the shock of diagnosis wears off, old behaviors, dynamics, and former roles return. Much of what is discussed in support groups revolves around the hurt and angry feelings caregivers have about this. That is not to say all families act in this manner, but it seems many do.

It is very important for caregivers to know when, where, and how they can expect support. This clarification, as awkward as it may be, must be made because it will free caregivers from spending time wishing things were different, and allow them to direct their energies to the necessary tasks of being a caregiver.

I am a proponent of family meetings where issues are laid out, expectations aired, everyone has an opportunity to be heard, and caregiving preferences and timetables are discussed. This usually encompasses many meetings, but it does away with wishful thinking and mind-reading. A monthly meeting or text update to all involved is a good precedent to establish.

Our children have been a source of comfort in entirely different ways that reflect their own unique abilities. Our son, Brian, who lives across the country in California, is a wonderful supporter and listener. He doesn't hesitate to point out something I don't see or may have missed. This is always done in a kind and constructive manner.

When we visit, he always plans special things to do, and makes sure the visit is a respite for me. His love for his father shines through in his actions and responses to his father. His heartbreak is also apparent, and I am well aware he struggles with what is happening and the inevitable loss of his father. I am his mother, and like all mothers, I want to fix it. This is one time my powers as a mother fail me.

Later when I transferred my husband to California, Brian stopped and visited him every day on his way to work or back. This brought great comfort to my husband, and to this day Brian will tell you how happy he is that he had that time to be with his father, even as painful as it was at times.

Our daughter, Laura, who lives in Alabama, is also a source of comfort, different in her own unique way and style. She, too, loves her father and it is clear her heart is breaking. Upon diagnosis, she became driven to make sure he would have a grandchild, so both would have an opportunity to know and love each other. Two of our most wonderful gifts are our darling granddaughters, Maddie and Lauren. The love I feel for them is so intense, and the appreciation of their arrival at this time in our life only adds to those feelings. I have found children to do remarkably well with people suffering from Alzheimer's. Their innocence, open hearts, and unconditional love make them natural allies.

Within the family unit, it can be too easy to feel disappointed, and caregivers must be on guard to make sure this doesn't happen. That's why open, honest communication, along with family meetings and updates is so important. If you are quick to label a behavior as uncaring, your own feelings can turn into disappointment and resentment.

It must be remembered, that although they are adults, children often have a very difficult time witnessing the decline of their parent. It is also important to remember that they have lives of their own with all that brings.

It is equally as important to remember that each family member adapts according to his/her own personality. It is not a good idea to put a family member in the middle of a disappointment or hurt or ask to take sides. No matter what your frustration is, placing someone in this tenable situation does not motivate anyone to want to help. I've witnessed families broken down, right at the point when they are most needed to be a conducive unit, because such behavior resulted in estrangement. It is smart to remember that most family members are doing the best they can. And when they are not, hard as it may be, let it go, move on, and stay focused on what is important.

Friends

When I think of friends an old song comes to mind: "Make new friends but keep the old, one is silver and the other gold." I cannot stress enough the importance of making new friends, while keeping the old. Aside from the fact that it is inevitable that some old friends will disappear (this has nothing to do with you, but is a reflection of them), new friends have the unique ability to offer a different kind of friendship.

> Some friends disappeared into the night, but with the passing of time, I came to accept it as a part of the human condition.

They will be the friends who GET IT, who support you, and make you not feel so alone. Nothing is more comforting than someone who truly gets you.

I used to, in the beginning, be annoyed with some friends who disappeared into the night, but with the passing of time, I have come to accept it as a part of the human condition. I remember one hilarious moment watching a friend hide out in produce, while I was grocery shopping. The only time I found it annoying is when I am about to become someone's cause or someone falls all over me with "How can I help?" never to be seen again.

Support Group Friends

Joining a support group is an absolute necessity, but the problem often lies in finding the right one. Don't give up if the first one is not right for you, or the next or the next, because there will be a support group out there with your name on it, just waiting for you. The value of being in a group, aside from the wonderful support and knowing you are not alone with

> It is smart to remember that most family members are doing the best they can. And when they are not, hard as it may be, let it go, move on, and stay focused on what is important.

this disease, is that you have the opportunity to learn from those who have gone before you, commiserate with those who are where you are, and welcome and help those who are just starting out. It is a safe haven where you can talk about all your feelings, without fear of judgment.

This is another reason to be in a support group: These folks walk the walk, and platitudes are not a part of their vocabulary. I am always amazed at what is laid on the table during these meetings, with never an eyebrow raised in question of disdain. This is the best support you can receive.

A support group also offers caregivers an opportunity to watch as others struggle with issues that aren't presently theirs, but may be down the road. Consider going online if there is no support group in your area or if getting out of the house is difficult. Please don't miss out on this wonderful life-saving resource. I can guarantee you, this will make your caregiver role easier and sustain you along the journey.

weekend away

We had a weekend away in Boston,
  with the children, who had not seen their dad since
  Christmas.
  He was perfect, symptom free, and on his very best
  behavior.
  Almost like a child with company, suddenly the report
  that I had conveyed rang less true.
  And nicely, ever so nicely, it was suggested I might be
  exaggerating.
  Who was I to argue?
  Grateful for just a normal weekend, grateful for the
  respite, however brief in nature.
  And knowing, when they are ready, they will see.
  It will be many months later before they finally see
  what I see.

brief moments

They've taken him out in the ocean with them for a swim,
these children of mine who struggle with the inevitable.
They circle around him, protective and loving, like he
once did with them.
And I lay back on the chaise, close my eyes and feel
the warmth of the sun.
For a few brief moments, he is not my responsibility.
I luxuriate in the belief that life is like it once used to be.

sigh

Not just occasionally, but all the time.
That's what my children tell me.
It seems I sigh.
Surely they are wrong, I don't sigh, at least not all
the time.
But now with my new awareness, I catch myself sighing.
How could I have been so unaware?
When did I slip into this despicable habit?

I sigh, it seems, long mournful sighs when things don't
go my way,
when I am tired, when I am disappointed, even when I
am at rest.
I start to apologize, but my children will not hear of it.
They tell me it is good to sigh; it is healthy.
When did they become so smart, I wonder, as I let out
a long sigh.

talk over him

We talk over him as if he were not there, our daughter
the first to notice,
the first to point it out, adding she felt badly.

We talk over him, staring at the space above his head,
at least, that's how a longtime friend described it,
admitting sheepishly she found herself growing
impatient with him at times.
We talk over him at family functions, already rambunctious
in nature, as if he were no longer a part, secretly
wondering if it is true, dreading the day when it will be.

I talk over him, as if he was not there, making all the
decisions unilaterally,
and holding conversations in my head.

We talk over him.
All aware of what we are doing, saddened by our actions,
frustrated by our thwarted attempts to include him,
embarrassed by taking the low road, when clearly the
high road is called for.

I talk over him, as if he
was not there, making all
the decisions unilaterally,
and holding conversations
in my head.

special gift

We await the birth of our first grandchild, coming at
a much needed time in our life.
There will be other grandchildren, but none like this
child.
Special in so many ways, bringing hope into a life short
on hope,
and sustaining me through this ordeal.
This special child, whose development will parallel my
husband's losses.

We will celebrate as one learns to walk, mourn as the
other forgets.
We will be filled with joy as this special child says her
first words, and
sadness as the other utters his last words.
We will look to the future with one, and remember the
past with the other.
Such perfect timing, this special child and my husband;
companions on a journey with different destinations.

my daughter and I

On a recent trip to visit my mother-in-law in Maine,
   the purpose being to introduce her to her great-
   granddaughter,
   my daughter and I shared a hotel room, while my
   husband stayed with his mother.
   We put the baby in the crib, turned off the lights so
   she could sleep, and I slipped down to
   the bar for two Sea Breezes.

My daughter crawled into bed next to me, reminiscent
   of the days when she was little.
   The room was dark, expect for the glow of the moon
   through the window.
   The conversation was soft, not to wake the baby,
   allowing the lapping of the waves against
   the shore to be heard.
   The atmosphere was reassuring, the darkness bringing
   with it a sense of safety,
   setting the stage for questions never before asked to
   come forth.

She shared a concern that she and her brother were at
   risk for inheriting the disease, her sadness over seeing
   her father's decline, the unfairness of it all, and then in
   what must have been a leap of faith,
   she asked the question that had been weighing on her
   mind: "Would I leave her father?"
   I told her the truth:
   The answer was NO, but at some point, I would need
   to seek alternative care.
   She said she understood, for which I was greatly relieved.

We finished our drinks, feeling like two school girls on an
   adventure—
   both having taken risks and survived.

shell

"Dad is just a shell of himself," my son tells me during
   a recent visit home,
   having not seen him in months.
   I feel the words forming as my defenses and denial
   kick in.
   We can still have conversations, go to dinner, enjoy
   movies, limited as this all may be,
   we can still do this.

But nothing comes out. I remain silent, transfixed by
   the sadness on my son's face.
   He is losing a father long before he should; I cannot
   imagine that pain.
   I am desperately holding onto any semblance of
   normality.
   He is struggling to come to terms with an unbearable
   reality.
   Through his eyes, I see what I have not wanted to see.
   I wonder what he sees through my eyes.

my son and I

My son and I share this new relationship.
The boundaries not quite worked out, still a little
awkward.
Over the phone, he answers my computer questions,
insisting they would end if I simply signed up for a
course. Like I have time for that.
He advises me on which credit card is the best, tells
me my cell phone plan is way too high,
listens to me when I am weary, never judging, just
listening.

He urges me to move to California, where he could offer
more help.
But he respects my decision that I am not ready yet
and does not push.
It seems like just yesterday I had all the answers.
When did the tables get turned?

watch

I watch him, our son, as he watches over his father,
very protective, very patient.
"This way, Pops, not that way."
"Let me get that for you."
"Let me help you."

It was only yesterday they were often locked, going
head-to-head, toe-to-toe.
Now he tells his father that he is his role model and
always has been,
bringing tears to my eyes.
How quickly old hurts, resentments are put aside.
My son is now the one leading.
He has become a father to his father.

my heart

My heart had been locked, bolted down, shut and secure.
   Worn out by life's travails: passing of a parent,
   impact of downsizing, daughter's diagnosis of
   idiopathic kidney disease,
   death of a pet, and my husband's diagnosis of early-
   onset Alzheimer's.

My heart was safe, on permanent hiatus, protected from
   random assaults.
   My illusions had all been shattered.
   A conscious decision made to hold life at arm's length.
   And I did just that, until I held my first grandchild in
   my arms.

Then my heart opened, welcoming in joy, and making
   room for hope and new beginnings.

maddie

In the midst of darkness and devastation, Maddie came
into the world.
Our first grandchild surprised me with the intensity of
feelings
she aroused in what I thought was a heart worn down,
no longer capable of seeing the light, feeling the
warmth.

She opened my heart immediately and slowly, all at the
same time.
Month by month delighting in her antics, responding to
her reaching out to the world,
as she grew into toddlerhood, awakening us both to
the infinite possibilities and pleasures of the world.

She gave to me the gift I needed and only she could
give. I saw the world through her eyes and fell in love
with life again.

lauren

My second granddaughter, so different from the first.
Less intense, just happy to be here, content to watch
her big sister.
Beaming a ray of sunshine with her smile so contagious.
I pick her up and she responds, smiling and cooing.
How nice it is to be responded to, I'd almost forgotten.
What a gift this bundle of happiness with her small
arms around my neck,
reminding me of the warmth of touch and the
importance of being loved.
How fortunate I am to be her grandmother.

liam

My darling grandson, who arrived four years after
my husband's death,
expanding and thrilling our family simultaneously.
A happy child blessed with boundless energy and
enthusiasm, delighting us to no end,
reminding us of his grandfather, by sharing some of
the same interests,
exhibiting the same curiosity.

How his grandfather would have loved him; how he
would have loved his grandfather.
Two people destined never to meet by a fate that
seems so cruel.
Still two people who will never know each other, but
will forever be connected by love.

Our first grandchild surprised me with
the intensity of feelings she aroused in
what I thought was a heart worn down,
no longer capable of seeing the light,
feeling the warmth.

message to friends

Do not romanticize this disease or speak to me about it
   being a gift.
   There is nothing romantic about this illness and the
   gifts come at too high a price.
   Do not speak to me about the quality of life, for it is a
   quality greatly redefined,
   and one that would be foreign to the person he or she
   once was.
   Do not speak to me about the Zen of Alzheimer's or
   people returned to a kinder,
   gentler state, as the cost to the soul is too great.
   To serve up platitudes is an insult.

Instead, listen to what I and other caregivers say.
   We are the ones who deal with it on a 24/7 basis. Sit
   with us and understand our plight as we see it, not as
   you see it.
   Be still with your own discomfort. You don't need to
   rush in to save us both,
   or offer trivial suggestions under the guise of caring.
   Just be there with me; nothing more is needed.

There are tears, but laughter
too, along with a sense of
not being alone, and relief
that finally someone gets it.

friends before alzheimer's

To my friends before Alzheimer's,

you mean so much to me, more than you will ever know.

Yet, somewhere along the way, our relationship has shifted.

Often I find myself carrying the conversation for two, working, at the same time, not to burden you with my problems, well aware you have your own.

Suddenly, it seems, our presence has become a problem in need of a solution.

We really don't fit in anymore.

We have become half of a couple, a reminder that this could happen to you, too.

A reminder of your own mortality.

Then there is the ambivalence I feel.

I see your lives stretching out before you, while ours is shrinking.

The talk of travel that had been promised for our retirement years,

the excitement of this new stage in our lives,

the privilege of a shared history,

the warmth of being a couple, a future going forward.

I am well aware I no longer have that.

I feel happiness for you and wish you well.

But, I feel sadness for us and sorrow for what tomorrow brings.

support group

Sitting in my support group, a safe haven where we
    share stories, unload our burdens,
    discuss our concerns, support each other, I feel at
    home.
    There are tears, but laughter too, along with a sense
    of not being alone, and
    relief that finally someone gets it.

This is what binds us together. This is what gives us the
    strength for another day.
    The room is safe and warm, reflecting the genuineness
    of its inhabitants.
    Outside it is raining—a torrential downpour that shows
    no signs of letting up—a reflection
    of the inward part of us that we keep hidden, except
    for the times we come together.

mirror image

She is new to our support group, this woman who
    speaks of her husband's recent
    diagnosis in the most optimistic of terms.
    Positive a cure is just around the corner, relying on just
    the right combination
    of vitamins and antioxidants to stave off the disease,
    planning lots of wonderful events, meticulously
    scheduling his days designed
    to keep his mind sharp, religiously surfing the internet
    to ensure his treatment is state-of-the-art,
    convincing herself this will really work, giving them the
    home court advantage.

I smile to myself as she speaks.
    Once I was in her place, a mirror image.

strong

"You are so strong." A sentiment I hear much too often,
   and it grates on my fragile nerves.
   What does it mean? I haven't fallen to pieces (yet)?
   Why is it said? A reassurance? And if so, for whom?
   I am no stronger than any of the other caregivers
   coping with this disease—
   members who comprise my support group, caregivers
   who have gone before me,
   or those who will be in my place someday.

We all do what it takes, discover inner resources we
   never knew we had,
   take it day by day, and live in the moment.
   What other choice is there?
   But then I realize I am strong; we are all strong, made
   possible by necessity.
   We made the choice and became strong.
   And now I hear the remark as it was meant to be heard.

questions without answers

My friend from my support group who threw me a lifeline,
   who knew what it was like,
   against whom I measured my progress and the
   progress of the disease, has had a stroke.
   How can that be? Isn't she too young?
   Isn't that a disease of the elderly?
   Isn't that what we said about Alzheimer's?

why?

I thought I was past the anger, had come to terms
  with the disease,
    but now I feel the anger swell, taking on a new
    freshness, a life of its own.
    This is not the same anger, but new and different.

How can my friend of 52 be lying in a hospital bed
  from a stroke?
    She who has given up her life to be a caregiver to
    her husband,
    borne all the responsibilities to a man no longer a
    husband, let alone a companion.
    Is he the reason she is lying in that bed?

How were we to know?
    What should we have looked for?
    Why didn't we pay more attention to our support
    group leader's plea for us to take care of ourselves?
    She seemed to have reached a level of acceptance,
    a peace.
    But all along a time bomb was silently ticking, just
    waiting to go off.
    Why must this disease claim two?

**Why didn't we pay more attention
to our support group leader's plea
fro us to take care of ourselves?**

bets

Jokingly we place bets, wagers of sort, these support
   group ladies of mine,
      most of whom have been together from the beginning.
   We place bets in our minds, occasionally giving voice
   to it,
      while eyeing the new member whose husband is
      moving rapidly along,
      while for some of us, the decline is moving inch by
      inch, year by year.

> **Black Humor is a caregiver's
> tool, designed to assuage our
> guilt at having such dreadful
> thoughts.**

A blessing in the *Beginning Stage,* not so much in
   Middle, and a curse by *Final Stage.*
   Like sports fans, we tally up the odds, silently placing
   our bets.
   These are our husbands, fathers of our children, our
   partners in life.
   Still we can't keep from placing our bets, reminding
   ourselves Black Humor is a caregiver's tool, designed
   to assuage our guilt at having such dreadful thoughts.

ultimate relief?

One of my support group friend's husband died.
   We, the ladies in the group, received the news with
   mixed reactions.
   It seems it was much too soon, but on the other hand
   fortunate for both of them.
   Nothing our support group friend would not have said
   or thought if places were reversed.
   After all, we'd discussed the issue many times before
   and often wondered why those
   who went before us were not feeling set free.

But the new widow, as outspoken and honest as ever,
   warned us not to tell her it was a blessing
   or that she'd been spared, because now she knew
   what the widows who went before her knew.
   What we all found so in opposition to our collective
   tiredness and lonely hearts—
   this is a terrible loss even is spite of years of
   caregiving, running the entire show, interacting,
   only with a shadow of what once was the person
   we loved,
   and achingly longing for relief in our most desolate
   moments,
   it seems what we thought would turn out to be the
   ultimate relief, turns out to not be so.

good intentions

It seems they all start out with good intentions, these
   ladies in my support group.
   Each declaring their undying devotion:
   No husband of theirs will ever go into an assisted living
   memory care unit or a nursing home.
   And I watch with fascination their devotion, their loyal-
   ty, wondering where mine is, as they declare, they will
   keep their husbands home, bring in outside help, turn
   the family room into a bedroom,
   the house into a fortress.

Good intentions abound, sincere and from the heart,
   but one by one as the disease progresses,
   these good intentions start to break down.
   Thoughts turn to possibilities of assisted living with
   memory care, as physical demands increase,
   fatigue sets in, and the resolve behind the good
   intentions wavers,
   as one by one these ladies in my support group grow
   wearier with each passing day.

CHAPTER 12

This I Know

I would like to think I have grown wiser with the years, but the plain truth is I have grown wiser with the disease.

As we transitioned from *Beginning Stage* to *Middle Stage*, I congratulated myself on how far we had come, and how well we had done. This transition from *Middle Stage* to the *Final Stage* brings no such congratulations, because I am well aware what the next stage brings. This will be a time of very difficult and intense decisions that will have to be made. And this will be the final good-bye, with all the sadness, heartache, and mixed feelings it brings.

During both *Beginning* and *Middle Stages*, I lost my husband slowly, day by day, month by month, and year by year. Yet, he was still able to communicate, enjoy small pleasures, and retain an essence of his former self. I am well aware this will not be the case going forward. I have prepared myself, hopefully, for the day when he truly will be just a shell of his former self, and for the dreaded and cruel time when he will no longer recognize me. I have been told at this point, that just being present is enough. I hope that turns out to be true.

While we still have the most difficult and, perhaps, longest part of the journey ahead, I do feel less alone these days, grown more aware of the cycle of life with its beginnings and endings, learned to sit with my feelings, and feel more capable of handling what this *Final Stage* will bring. Still it is with a sense of sadness that I say good-bye to *Middle Stage*, a stage where glimmers of sameness would arise, bringing back times of no worry and looking forward to tomorrow.

change of heart

I use to be judgmental, full of pronouncements,
    before the illness.
    Case in point: my mother's friend, five years into the
    second marriage,
    who could no longer care for her husband diagnosed
    with dementia.
    In my infinite wisdom, I concluded her behavior was
    typical "second wife syndrome."

I listened to women in my support group,
    whose husbands were further along than mine,
    elaborate on how they could no longer tolerate the
    mess, or stand the strain.
    And in my infinite wisdom, I thought, "What's the big
    deal?"

I use to think self-sacrifice was what marriage was
all about.
    So my career, my life, took back stage, despite it being
    the era of consciousness raising.
    And in my infinite wisdom, dismissed the message.

I use to think being female made me responsible for
everyone and everything,
    a belief indoctrinated from the moment of birth.
    And in my infinite wisdom, being the good girl, I dared
    not question it.
    I use to give literal interpretation to the vow "In sickness
    and in health"—
    even if the cost meant my health, too.
    So in my then infinite wisdom, I vowed no spouse of
    mine would go into a nursing home.

I would like to think I have grown wiser with the years,
    but the plain truth is I have grown wiser with the
    disease.
    No longer will I assume responsibility for everyone and
    everything.
    Or judge others whose course or choices are different
    than mine.
    Or sacrifice my health and sanity.
    The price is too high.

There are two people in this equation
    and this illness dips the scales so drastically
    that if I am to survive, if I am to be of any help to him,
    I have to give up my judgments,
    lay my infinite wisdom aside,
    and open myself up to new ways of being.

new definition of quality

How can there be quality of life for someone afflicted
    with Alzheimer's?
    Is the question not an oxymoron
    when one has been robbed of the most precious gifts
    of memory and mind?
    When days are locked into endless repetition of
    questions and phrases, years mirror one another,
    and the progression continues its steady decline?

How can there be quality of life for the caregiver when
    the caregiving hours increase,
    the progression of the disease marches on,
    the home is turned into a fortress,
    and the caregiver becomes a prisoner,
    with burnout the inevitable conclusion?

Those were the questions I wrestled with when first
    faced with the impact of this disease,
    questions that mirrored my feelings and beliefs.
    But over the years, I have had to challenge my
    responses to these questions,
    come to terms with my conflicting feelings,
    factor into the equation the needs of both parties,
    and redefine the definition of quality of life.

And I have come to understand
    that there will come a time for me to let go,
    to place my husband in a different environment,
    where his functional abilities are maximized and his
    independence promoted.
    Where he will have options and his dignity preserved,
    so setting a table becomes a source of pride, not a chore.
    Waving his arms and legs in a group dance, not silly,
    but meaningful.
    Lingering over memories of the past, not simply a way
    to pass time, but a way to stay connected.

And I will need to remind myself at those moments that
quality, like beauty, is in the eye of the beholder.
And if I can let go of what was, accept what is, and my
new role,
work through the accompanying sadness and loss,
be secure in the knowledge that I have done all I could,
then I believe peace will follow,
bringing with it a new definition of quality of life.

needs

I will weather this storm and make it through, like those
who have gone before me did.
I have gone so far, so much into the darkness of the
night and soul, with more still to come.
I will need family even more now,
the joy of my grandchildren to bring me respite from
the storm,
the love of my children to anchor me,
the understanding and guidance of our doctors who
partner with us in this disease,
friends to see me through and remind me not all is lost,
my support group to lean on and share the feelings
weighing heavy on my heart.

I will need to be strong for myself,
find a new identity or way of being in the world.
I will need to draw on the strengths that have gotten
me this far,
and I will need to remember, even in the darkness of
night, morning comes.

the new me

The new me is alive and kicking, not so different from
the old.
After all, we each have a core from which we operate.
But the new me puts up with less, cuts to the point
quicker,
understands and applies the meaning of choice,
and is not driven by duty, unless it is defined by me.
The new me has a softness, an appreciation of the
plight of others,
and a respect for the trials and tribulations of life.

The new me is less judgmental of others and content to
let people be who they are,
and careful not to get tangled up where I don't belong
or in a way that does not serve me.

The new me understands that selfish is not always bad,
and that I have needs that also must be addressed and
met.
The new me has cleaned closets, both real and literal,
learned to travel lighter,
appreciate the moment, and feel gratitude for the
good in my life.

The new me is ready for what is coming next.

The new me has a softness, an appreciation of the plight of others, and a respect for the trials and tribulations of life.

unguarded moment

Sometimes in quiet moments, caught off guard,
the magnitude of it all overwhelms me.
I feel my body stiffen, my heartbeat accelerates.
A growing sense of uneasiness threatens to overtake
me as I wonder how I will survive what is yet to come.
Then I look back and see how far I have come.
Then I know.

trust

We are cruising, a new experience, surrounded by miles
of ocean with no land in sight.
Each day brings the same horizon.
Each evening is surrounded by pitch black—not even
the moon to light its way,
leaving us without bearings, or so it seems.
I must trust the ship to find its way to port, as I must
trust myself to find my way to tomorrow.

fine

On rare occasions, when people inquire how I am, most
often the inquiry being about my husband,
I reply, "Fine." The expected response to this social
question.
But I am fine, having railed against the disease, the
injustice of it all, of what it did to our lives, our family.
All the pieces are still there, just the puzzle no longer
connects.
But still I am fine, having made the necessary
adjustments, rearranged our lives,
and come to terms with a disease that steals
something from everyone it touches.

terrain traveled

This is not a journey measured by miles, scenic signposts,
  Kodak moments, or selfies.
    Yet, we have traveled far from the safety of our former
    existence, to strange and unfamiliar places,
    met with people once foreign to us,
      covered terrain that was unfamiliar, often treacherous
      and never lost our way.

Though the journey is far from over, the terrain has
  become familiar, the path less daunting.
    But we know not to be lulled into a false sense of
    security,
      for it can change without a moment's notice.

How strange to be traveling this journey, unplanned and
  undesired.
    Still, in many ways, rewarding.
    People we have met have shown us the meaning of the
    word, "courageous."
    This disease has challenged our once complacent
    values, realigned our priorities,
      introduced us to a different world, offered us another
      path to travel,
      and shown us, most importantly, how the beauty of the
      human spirit illuminates the way.

three

Final Stage

CHAPTER 13

Transitioning to Final Stage

My caregiving skills were running on empty, and adding to my compassion fatigue was the knowledge that Final Stage encompasses the potential for some very intense decisions.

Having successfully navigated the *Beginning* and *Middle Stages*, I knew as we approached the end of *Middle Stage* that the direction of caregiving would become increasingly more difficult. What I did not know was how that difficulty would manifest itself and what my response would be.

As the disease slowly edged its way toward *Final Stage,* I was well aware it could encompass many years, so I became more diligent about recording my thoughts, lest I forget them. Forgetting, it seems, is just not limited to those with dementia. "Senior Moments" for me were now becoming more common, and I was well aware overload and stress can wreak havoc with one's memory.

What surprised and concerned me most was the increasing difficulty I experienced in remembering our life before Alzheimer's. I was not alone as this concern was becoming a frequent topic in my support group. Many a session was spent discussing how hard it was to connect with "what was" as we caregivers became more and more immersed in the daily "what is."

Experts in the field warn caregivers that *Final Stage* can very often be the longest. I know one thing for sure ... it is the saddest. *Beginning Stage* carries with it time still available to do things, the promise of hope, and a possible cure. During this stage the caregiver's role is one of companion and life can still proceed, almost, as before. By *Middle Stage*, reality really sets in as duties and responsibilities increase markedly, along with feelings of fatigue and loneliness. The role of companion has now changed to one of caregiver.

Final Stage carries no promises, no hope, as any leftover illusions give way to finality. For some it is a silent prayer that the person being cared for and the caregiver will be spared a long drawn out decline, along with the accompanying feelings of guilt for such thoughts; for others, it can be a time of holding on with fierce intensity. At this juncture, the caregiver has now become a custodian.

As I approached the end of *Middle Stage*, I did so with an increased sense of exhaustion. My husband was disappearing before my eyes, leaving very little of who he had been to connect with. The sense of sadness was overwhelming as I grappled with the reality of what was coming next.

My caregiving skills were running on empty, and adding to my compassion fatigue was the knowledge that *Final Stage* encompasses the potential for some very intense decisions. From the distance of the past two stages, these decisions don't seem so daunting, but as one gets closer to *Final Stage*, the impact of the job as decision maker for another's life can send a caregiver into a paralysis or, at least, a tailspin.

It is my belief, based on the feedback I have received from caregivers through support groups I've been in, through dialogue with audience members when I speak, and through simply being a witness to the disease, that caregivers can come perilously close to losing themselves at this point. This is not surprising given the inordinate number of months and years that caregiving can encompass. Trying to carve out a separate life—along with the dichotomy of staying connected while letting go—is the major task for caregivers during final stage.

> Now I knew I had to really start looking to my future and my needs, as well as my husband's, if I wanted any life when my job as caregiver was over.

At this juncture, I was increasingly aware of how much my life had changed. Shortly after placing my husband in assisted living, I noticed how still both my house and life had become. In the beginning the stillness was a welcomed relief and I cherished it, but now it was becoming something that was making me uneasy. My job, my identity, most of my interests, along with many friends, had disappeared, as Alzheimer's consumed more and more of my time.

My own health had suffered and I realized I was not taking good care of myself. I hadn't even noticed because it happened slowly over the years as result of caregiving. Now I knew I had to really start looking to my future and my needs, as well as my husband's, if I wanted any life when my job as caregiver was over. It was during this period I was diagnosed with early stage endometrial cancer, which I believe to this day, was brought about by stress.

It was as if all the forces came together during this period of my life. My elderly parents, who were living in Florida, had now begun to have serious medical issues that required my help. I found myself on a flight to Florida about once a month for a week's stay, while I took them to doctors and helped out as best as I could.

Final Stage carries no promises, no hope, as any leftover illusions give way to finality.

As I began the *Final Stage* of our journey, I was acutely aware of what needed to be done for my husband, and what needed to be done for me. I was also aware that I could not do this alone, and that I now needed to call on more resources in a greater capacity. I knew it would not be easy, and I would have times of great conflict, but I knew I could do this, sustained by how far I had come, the kindness of others, and my own faith and understanding. I had not given up, nor had I surrendered; I'd simply made peace with the situation.

Throughout *Beginning* and *Middle Stage*, I recorded my thoughts and reflections on caregiving with great ease. By the almost end of *Final Stage*, it became a chore to do so. When visiting my husband and seeing him constantly sleeping or curled into a ball, unable to utter any words, the visual of that was enough. I simply did not want to have a written record. It takes strength and fortitude to see someone in a situation like this on every visit. Not surprisingly, visits greatly decline during this period—often referred to as "drive-by" visits. It is a shame because we have no way of knowing what awareness or feelings an Alzheimer's patient has at that point. I could not leave my husband all alone at this time, but it often took great will to get through the doors of the assisted living facility. I know he would have done it for me, and I often reminded myself of that.

status

I am married, but I am not married.
> I am not widowed, but, in many ways, I am.
> What am I now that I am suspended in between these
> two categories?
> A married widow, perhaps.
> I wear my wedding band out of habit.
> I honor my vows out of respect.
> I am a caregiver bereft of what constitutes a marriage.

And as the years pass, the memory of what was fades
> with not much to replace it.
> I need a new status to reflect my situation of straddling
> two worlds.
> And so I found it ... a beautiful ring with two circles of
> small diamonds connected ever so briefly, representing
> our union ... connected but separate.

not real

In the *Beginning Stage*, when everything seemed alien
> and made no sense,
> when surely it was all a mistake, a terrible
> misunderstanding, it just was not real.

In *Middle Stage*, where he was still there, just not quite
> there, and I was stretched beyond my limits, it was real.

In *Final Stage*, impacted by the atrocity of watching him
> disappear before my eyes, saddened by a life forever
> altered, there was no room for denial.
> It was real ... very, very real.

photos

I look at pictures in the old family albums and on the
   computer, trying hard to remember the past.
   The good times seem so elusive now, even imaginary.
   Who are those youngsters in the wedding album?
   Thank God, they didn't know then what I know now.
   And if they were privy to such information, what would
   they have done?

I scan photos taken over the years searching for clues.
   At what moment did it start to go wrong?
   Is it here in the photo where he looks lost and distant?
   Or here where he clearly is not himself?
   I look at the photos and see no evidence of the future
   we now know.
   The camera clicked and all was well.
   Suspended between present and past,
   I close the album, leaving our innocence intact.

> **He is lost in a world where
> no one can reach him, no
> one can love him, and no one
> can make him feel safe.**

reminded

I am reminded that darkness does not just come at the
   end of the journey, with its melancholy sadness of the
   inevitable,
   when the situation can seem almost untenable,
   when prolonged suffering is more than one can bare.
   I am reminded of that sitting here in my support group,
   after an absence, listening to members at the beginning
   of their journey, suddenly thankful I have traveled these
   miles and survived.

I sense now with more clarity and experience behind
   me, the grip that darkness can have at its inception in
   Beginning Stage:
   in the questions asked and withheld,
   in the family members unable to rally or cope,
   in the realization that life will never be the same,
   in the fear for the future,
   in the often frozen stance taken, as we prepare for
   tomorrow.

Once I, too, was afraid of darkness.
   Fought it,
   hid from it,
   denied it,
   ran from it.
   But now I understand and no longer fear darkness. Its
   grip has lessened over the years.
   Now I sit, instead, with darkness, listening quietly for
   the message,
   understanding full well it is a necessary part of the
   journey.
   Knowing that birth and death are the cycles of life, and
   after darkness, the light returns.

waiting

Waiting is what caregivers do.

How can caregivers wait you ask, when their life is full of nonstop activities, routines, responsibilities?

But wait they do, and it is a different kind of waiting from what they have known before.

Caregivers wait from the moment of diagnosis.

Some in shock, some in fear, some in denial, some in disbelief, waiting to see what is next and how they will cope.

Caregivers wait in *Middle Stage*, when the shock has worn off and a semblance of hope is still present, waiting to see what this new stage will bring and how they will cope. Some still in crisis mode, some in coping mode, some having made peace.

> **Caregivers wait to be set free from this collective nightmare they share.**

Caregivers wait in *Final Stage*, for the final days to come.

Some in exhaustive states, some in resignation, some in relief, some in grief, waiting to see if they can make it through the saddest stage.

Caregivers wait to be set free from this collective nightmare they share.

Some ready, some not sure, some pointed toward tomorrow, others holding onto today; they wait wondering what life will bring.

Caregivers wait in each stage—a natural part of the caregiving process—giving them time to recoup, process their feelings, and prepare.

conflicting emotions

I want to run, to go away—some place, far, far away.
  A one-way ticket is all I need; travel light and never
  look back.
  Reinvent myself and start over … busy every minute.
  No downtime—out with friends every waking moment
  doing, doing, doing.
  No time for thoughts of what lies ahead.
  Manic, frantic, frenetic.

No, I want to hide, nest, and cocoon.
  Hibernate till it's all over, safe and secure in my own world.
  Not make any more decisions, responsible for only myself.

Who would have thought *Final Stage* could be so
  conflicting?
  It was supposed to come with some relief
  for my husband, who never would have wanted this
  existence,
  for my family, who find it increasingly difficult to weather.

But I was wrong … it is filled with finality,
  unrelenting sadness,
  difficult decisions,
  a barrage of conflicting emotions,
  along with the knowledge, this is really the end.

Who would have thought
this *Final Stage* could be
so conflicting?

my third child

Years ago we planned for our third child.
  Picked out names, made room in the house,
  entertained loving thoughts, but it never happened
  and we went on with our life.
  Years passed and while the sense of longing
  diminished, it never quite went away.
  Watch out what you wish for—that old adage, it seems,
  may be true.
  Suddenly, I have my third child or, at least, that's what
  it feels like.

mothering skills

How strange it is to dress my husband.
  Limbs seem to hang with no purpose or suddenly turn
  obstinate and rigid, as he stares straight ahead;
  the polar opposite of when I dress my grandchild.
  Her face eager with anticipation, her limbs supple and
  willing.

Will I ever get used to it?
  I doubt it.
  The strangeness of large body parts,
  the disconnected feeling—him from his body as I
  struggle to get him to cooperate, and me from the
  situation at hand.
  Then there's the negative chatter that dances through
  my mind while I brush his teeth, comb his hair, and
  toilet him, so he can start his day.
  Where have my mothering skills gone?

shared experience

My daughter and I exchange toileting tips these days.
   What is the best way?
   How does one keep her cool?
   Are constant reminders the solution?
   Should rewards be used? My granddaughter, it seems,
   is not cooperating, a situation quite familiar to me
   these days.

What insights can I offer her?
   Only that my granddaughter won't go off to college
   wearing diapers, and there is an end in sight.
   Otherwise, we are on the same page:
   sharing the same feelings,
   dealing with the same frustrations,
   reaching the end of the proverbial rope.

parallels

I watch my granddaughter learn as my husband regresses.
   Fascinated by her zest for life,
   discouraged by his apathy.
   Impressed by her new awareness of table manners,
   frustrated by his lack.
   Stimulated by her increasing vocabulary,
   annoyed by his increasing inarticulateness.
   Thrilled by her curious nature,
   depressed by his lack of awareness.
   Looking to the future with one,
   saddened for the future with the other.

bad mother/good mother

I am the bad mother.

Reduced to telling him NO, setting limits when his mind is made up and my patience has run out.

Sticking him in from of the TV for hours on end when I have grown weary of entertaining him.

Letting him eat far too much ice cream, when I know it is not good for his cholesterol.

Growing more and more impatient with his antics, no longer caring he cannot help it.

I am the good mother.

Overseeing the dreaded bath hour by making it fun.

Laying out his clothes and helping him get dressed.

Planning all his activities, driving him here and there.

Putting him first because there is no other choice.

Years ago I said good-bye to my mothering ways, but now, it seems, they have returned with a vengeance.

another sign

He took the dog for a walk ... just around the cul de sac;
  something he has done many times before, but this
  time he did not return.
  Minutes passed, in slow agony, with no sign of him or
  the dog.
  The neighborhood and adjoining streets scouted out in
  the car to no avail.
  Where could he have gone?
  Where could he possibly be?
  The neurologist warned me about this, but I thought it
  would never happen.
  Now it has ... another indicator of moving on has
  occurred.

I call the police and sheepishly describe my husband
  and dog.
  They are calm and assure me things will be fine.
  I am sure this is not their first time, but it is mine and I
  am feeling terribly remiss.

A police car arrives in my driveway and my husband,
  bursting with pride, announces his ride in the police
  car was so much fun.
  My dog appears unimpressed.

on script

"Who is that man? I don't like his face. Tell him to go
  away!" he yells while staring in the bathroom mirror.
  "There are men out there with guns," he barks at me,
  becoming more agitated minute by minute. "Close the
  drapes, now."
  "Throw that food away. It has poison in it," he declares,
  scowling at me.

Like an actress in a B-grade movie, following the script,
  I play my role.
  No reason to argue.
  No reason to be rational.
  No reason to become upset.
  Joining him on his journey, meeting him where he is,
  is the most expedient measure.

CHAPTER 14

Pre-Placement Days

At the same time as my husband slipped deeper and deeper into the darkness of the disease, I felt like I was on a parallel track.

"And then we go back to the United States." This was my husband's reply when I had finished outlining our itinerary for our stay in California during the upcoming holiday season. Six years into the illness, he was hovering perilously close to *Final Stage*. Mentally I ticked off the list of indicators:

✓ Incontinence

✓ Hallucinations

✓ Violence

✓ Wandering

At that point, he scored a "no" on the majority of these but shortly thereafter that would begin to change, along with increasing confusion and lack of functional abilities. His "stories" as I came to call them, never ceased to amaze or entertain me. Laced with bits of truth and intertwined with the outrageous, it made for some interesting stories. I came to learn that this behavior is referred to as confabulation and is a component of the disease.

My favorite story was what later lovingly became known as "The Airplane Story." My husband had done a lot of corporate travel in his day and, now, loved to reminisce about the time it was so foggy the captain asked him to roll down his window and help guide the plane to landing. We all smiled, but it was his granddaughters who saw the hero in him and asked him to tell the story over and over. Later down the road, the story was forgotten, along with his memory of having granddaughters.

As my husband connected more and more to the past, I connected less and less to it. So solidly stuck in the minutiae of day to day living, the past was something I had forgotten. It was as if I could no longer access the memories of the past or how he had once been. Many caregivers told me that it took a few years after the death of their spouse to reconnect and remember their spouses as they once had been.

Somewhere along the way I lost both my husband and myself. I use to wonder why caregivers, who recently lost their spouse, claimed they had no life. Before it made no sense to me, after all, they were finally free from the tediousness and heartbreak of this disease. But now I knew, now I saw how years of taking care of someone, putting yourself last, being stripped down to the basics, takes its toll.

This moment of revelation came to me as we perched precariously close to entering the *Final Stage* of our journey. I knew, then, that I had to start to get serious about planning for my life when my caregiving duties were over. Waiting till then would be too late.

The end of *Middle Stage* and the beginning of *Final Stage* ushered in an entirely new set of realities as the following changes had taken place:

- My husband could no longer shower unattended.

- He could no longer dress himself without my help.

- No longer could I point to the passenger side of the car, but now must lead him to it, put him in and buckle him up.

- He could no longer eat unattended, leaving me to cut up his food and help with the process.

- Trips to see the family were out of the question at this point.

- Verbally there was less and less interaction between us.

- And finally, the saddest of all, he no longer knew who his daughter was when she visited.

As the *Final Stage* approached, I knew the following decisions would soon be front and center:

- Placement in assisted living memory unit or keep him at home?
- Use of feeding tube?
- Would I change diapers?
- Continue on Aricept or not?
- Resuscitate or not?
- How aggressively to treat health issues?
- Bring in Hospice?
- What else?

As the *Final Stage* approached, I faced it with the reluctant martyrdom that often overcomes a long-term caregiver. I felt inured to the bleak existence and emotional pain that defined my life. The trappings of my previous life, along with my former identify were now gone. At the same time as my husband slipped deeper and deeper into the darkness of the disease, I felt like I was on a parallel track. One day I came across lines from Mary Oliver's poem, "The Journey" from her book, *New and Selected Poems:**

> but little by little,
> as you left their voices behind,
> the stars began to burn

At the same time as my husband slipped deeper and deeper into the darkness of the disease, I felt like I was on a parallel track.

through the sheets of clouds,
and there was a new voice
which you slowly recognized as your own,
that kept you company
as you strode deeper and deeper
Into the world,
determined to do
the only thing you could do—
determined to save
the only life you could save.

 Her poem literally saved my life and headed me in a new direction. It was as if clarity had finally entered my mind, and I knew then what the doctors, my support group leader, and friends were trying to tell me—this has gotten to be too much for me and it was time to start thinking about placement. I started the placement process, urged on by my support group leader who kept telling me, "You have no idea how exhausted you are." Like so many caregivers, I thought I could do it all and placement was for other people.

An interesting side note is soon after I placed my husband in assisted living memory unit for a two-week trial, the doctor called to tell me I had endometrial cancer. That two-week my trial became permanent; the cancer was successfully treated, and today I am fine. But, to this day, I believe that it was brought on by the unrelenting stress I was under and my disregard for my own health.

> **I had ignored my own health needs. I had simply ignored my own life.**

It was easier to put myself last as I was so busy with my husband's appointments. This is what happened with my yearly gynecological appointment; I simply forgot and paid the price.

This illness forced me into coming to terms with my needs and cemented the game plan and direction we would follow, going forward.

EXCERPT FROM A LETTER TO MY CHILDREN:

I have decided to write this letter versus email or text— even though much of its content has been discussed during our numerous phone calls and visits—because I feel it gives you an opportunity to think about it before you reply. I want to be clear that in no way, shape, or form am I looking for your approval; this is a decision only I, as primary caregiver and wife, can make.

I am planning on putting your father into assisted living memory care unit next month. He is showing more signs of confusion and there is increasing evidence that incontinence is around the corner. When I help dress Maddie, I can give her directions to follow, not so with your father. When I dress Lauren, she puts her arms up in anticipation, not so with your father.

When we go to dinner, there is no longer any conversation and I must cut his food. Vacations have become an ordeal and the thought exhausts me before I even begin.

I am increasingly coming closer and closer to my limitations and burnout. Sometimes, I feel like I don't know myself anymore. I know that this will be difficult to accept, but I believe your father will be happier in a place where everyone is in the same situation. He will have an opportunity for less stress in his life. I shall still visit him and continue to take care of him, I just won't be responsible for his day-to-day care.

I want to also take this time to remind you that there is a window of opportunity to still be with your dad. We never know when this window will close.

so sure

I was so sure I would put him in assisted living memory
   care unit when he wandered, became incontinent, and
   mixed up days and nights.
   The only one in my support group who had such plans,
   ironic now that I am the only one with a husband still
   at home.
   This decision is not as easy as I once thought it would be.

My freedom is nonexistent,
   my house has been turned into a fortress,
   all semblance of a life now gone as I have become a
   full-time custodian.
   And yet, I cannot turn over my role, it being far more
   painful, far more difficult than I ever imagined.
   Those who have gone before me, assured it is the best
   thing for both of us.
   And the proof is there in the eased lines etched on
   their faces, in their new demeanor.

So why am I stalling?
   Why am I holding on?
   Why am I looking for approval?
   Why is my analysis of the situation not sufficient?
   What happened to being so sure?

doubts

This is the most difficult thing I've ever had to do, one of
the most difficult decisions I've ever had to make.
I wonder if the sickening feeling in my stomach will be
with me forever as I question the wisdom of my decision.
How could I have been so sure this was the right thing
to do?
How did I sign admittance papers with such assurance?
I remember telling myself that all will be fine.

But now I am paralyzed by feelings of guilt and self-doubt.
I want to go back and undo it, but, at the same time,
I want to proceed.
Years later, when I had no choice but to place my mother
in a nursing home, these same doubts returned to
remind me—this is one of life's most difficult decisions.

angel

An elderly woman approaches me at the end of a talk
I have given.
She reaches out and takes my hand, holding it tenderly.
Her eyes, full of wisdom that only one who has been
on this journey, this path, can have.
And I know, intuitively, she is going to share something
profound, that she is an angel sent to me.
So I wait while she introduces herself, thanks me for
sharing my story.

Then she utters words I will never forget, words that
brought me such peace.
"Placing your husband in assisted living or a nursing
home will be harder than burying him."
I start to thank her, searching for the right words, but
she is gone, leaving me to wonder if I imagined it all.

promise

An illusionary promise of sorts is held out, almost like
   an olive branch,
   by members of my support group who have gone
   before me.
   They speak of love rekindled once a spouse is placed
   in assisted living or a nursing home.
   Of time now to enjoy him or her,
   having been released from the tediousness of 24/7
   caregiving.

They speak of positive memories that resurface,
   after years of lying dormant.
   But most importantly, they speak of an opportunity to
   close the final chapter by being able to reconnect with
   the emotions that gave substance and meaning to the
   union.

bedtime

Bedtime has once again become my favorite part of
   the day.
   Enticing me with its promise of peace,
   calling me to snuggle up, safely away from the cares of
   the day.
   I can feel it beckoning me, pulling like a magnet ...
   like the lure of an old bathrobe or comfortable pair of
   shoes.

My exhaustion mounting,
   my body succumbing till there is no longer an option.
   In the Beginning Stage weary from shock.
   In the Middle Stage weary from the increased
   responsibilities.
   Now in the Final Stage, weary from sadness of it all.

milestones

I thought it would happen when he became incontinent,
or wandered, or sun downed, or when behavioral
problems arose.
But it did not happen that way.
Days became longer and more difficult to get through.
Filled now with endless directions, orchestrating his
days and nights, along with bathing and feeding him.
My patience wore thin, till I no longer recognized
myself.
His confusion reached a level where he no longer knew
himself.
No longer was I a companion.
No longer was I a caregiver.
Now, it seemed, I had become a custodian,
watching over him 24/7.

I thought my decision to place him in an assisted living
memory unit would happen one day with a legitimate
reason to assuage my guilt.

Heads would nod in unison, after all incontinence,
wandering, sun downing, and behavioral problems
are accepted milestones, indicators that it is time for
placement.
But instead, I just wore out one day,
knowing I could no longer live a life for two.
Feeling like all caregivers feel ... if only I could have
done more.

more

What is more?

That elusive term that holds caregivers together in a
common bond.

What more could we do?

We've sacrificed, rearranged our lives, and restructured
our plans for the future.

But still we feel we could have done more.

What is it we could have done?

Why do we harbor regrets in the secret recesses of
our hearts?

We are "good enough" caregivers

doing the best we can with the situation we've been dealt.

There is no more we can do.

there is more

The small, secret voice tucked deep inside of me, where

I have buried it because I do not want to hear it,

taunts me even as I try not to pay attention.

The secret voice says, "There is more you can do and

you know it … you can take care of him and not place

him in assisted living."

What does the voice know of endless days, sleepless nights,

and no time for myself, exhaustion never known before?

If I listen to that voice, surely I will die before my

husband, who has years to go.

I have seen this firsthand and it is a valid Alzheimer's

caregiver statistic.

I must save myself, I must take care of myself; there is

no one else to do it.

And I am not abandoning my husband,

but I am abandoning that small, secret voice that holds

me prisoner.

hoped

I have set up the lights on the pine tree outside the living
room window, a feat in itself.
Gleaming white lights sparking against the falling snow.
Decorated the living room with candles burning
brightly in tune with Kenny G.
The tree perfectly decorated with past memories.
The wine has been poured,
the hors d'oeuvres baked.
A Currier & Ives Christmas even Martha Stewart would
be proud of.

It's just the two of us enjoying the magical moment of
the first snowfall of the season.
Outside it is a fairyland.
We sit in the living room warmed by the crackling fire,
but only I talk.
He sleeps, I am alone, except for the dog who has
become my constant companion and the male in
my life.

This is our last Christmas—at least the one he will be
present in any memorable manner.
I wanted everything to be perfect ... yet he sleeps
through it all, head bobbing along with Kenny G.
I sip my wine, feeling more alone than ever.
I should no longer be surprised or saddened.
This is our life, my life.
Yet, I hoped it could be different for just one night.

**What does the voice know of
endless days, sleepless nights,
and no time for myself, exhaustion
never known before?**

days before

The days before placement are the most difficult.
  Filled with second guessing,
  remorse, and guilt.
  Gotten through on auto pilot and angry outbursts.
  Thoughts of impending freedom from the tyranny of
  caregiving,
  along with tears that spring up out of nowhere.

Days that are reminiscent of adolescence and menopause,
  when emotions fluctuate moment by moment and life
  feels like a balancing act coming undone.
  Warm feelings one moment, negative thoughts the next.
  The bad parent, the good parent wrestle each other.
  No victory, for this decision carries no such promise.
  Bittersweet are the days before placement.
  Poignant in nature, testing the mettle of the human soul.

pretend

The phone rings, but I do not answer it.
  My cell calls out to be answered, but I let it be.
  It is another friend calling to wish me well, inquire if
  I need anything.
  Much appreciated but I want to be alone with my
  husband.

These final days belong to us.
  The last days we will live in our house of 30 years, the last
  days we will truly have together.
  These final days belong to just us and I guard them jealously.
  Even as he wanders aimlessly from room to room.
  Even as he is not present while he stands right next to me.
  I just want to pretend for these final days, final hours, that
  things are as they once were.

given

From the beginning, I have given you my life as you
gave me yours.

I have given you two children and supported you
through the years when you stumbled or wavered.

I have been by your side throughout this hideous
disease that has changed you from the man I knew to a
shadow of your former self.

I have given you more than I ever thought capable of,
glad to have the opportunity to do it.

But I cannot give you any more.

This situation now requires more than I am capable of.

I cannot give you what is left of my life; the cost being
my life.

I will not leave, I will be by your side in another capacity,
but it is time for me to save myself.

CHAPTER 15

Adjustment to Placement

I got into my own rhythm of visiting, and found various things to keep myself busy when I visited, sometimes simply just sitting and being present with him.

Adjustments have become a way of life for me over the years. It is almost as soon as one adjustment is completed, the next one is there ready to be made. Having reached the decision to place my husband in memory unit, I know had to adjust to my new life alone.

Shortly after placing him an assisted living memory care unit, I had surgery and I recovered quickly and within six months felt more like my old self. During some of the recovery time, I was unable to visit him. When I finally was able to visit him again, it made no impression on him. In many ways this freed me up to not hold on so tightly to the belief I had to go each and every day, even though I continued to do so, but l know it was out of choice, not obligation. That single belief was a blessing.

Over the years he was in assisted living memory care units, first two years in Connecticut, then two years in California, I could never quite shake the feeling that I should be visiting my parents in assisted living, not my husband. I got into my own rhythm of visiting, and found various things to keep myself busy when I visited, sometimes simply just sitting and being present with him. After two years at the first assisted living facility, it was suggested that he be moved to a nursing home due to his frequent falling, and that was not a viable option for him, nor for me.

I chose to move my husband to California because our son was there, and we had contacted a San Diego-based, world-renowned specialist about some new studies. My Connecticut neurologist assured me, when he heard what I was doing, the specialist would never have time to see us. But see us he did, and he added a valuable component to our treatment plan. It is this same neurologist (who I liked very much) that insisted it was an impossibility to transport an Alzheimer's patient at the stage my husband was, across the country.

My response was, "Watch me." At some point, it becomes very clear to caregivers what they can and cannot do, and much of the unwelcome advice goes right out the door.

The new assisted living memory care facility delivered a higher level of care and functioning to my husband. He loved the staff, engaged in activities, and sought out other residents. He had a good year and a half there, until his rapid decline in his last six months. The right assisted living facility is crucial. You may have to try a few before you find the right one; something you can't really know till you are there.

not so lucky this time

Years ago I lay on the surgeon's table,
  my breath held tightly in as I awaited the pathologist's
  report.
  Years later I lay in the pre-op room waiting for the
  anesthesiologist, wondering if the tumors were benign.
  I was lucky then and each time I promised life would
  be different—I would make time for myself.
  A promise broken but how was I to know what lay ahead.
  This time not so lucky, this time the dreaded diagnosis
  has come true.
  What-ifs run through my head, along with
  recriminations for not making time for myself.

I've seen firsthand Alzheimer's claim the caregiver before
  the one being cared for.
  That will not happen to me.
  This time I will keep my promise to myself.
  This time I have learned the lesson.
  It is time to place my husband in assisted living.
  No longer will excuses hold true, now I am the one
  who needs caregiving for the next six weeks.
  How strange, how sad, it took a cancer diagnosis to
  finally get me to see the light.

five miles

Today he is leaving his home of 30 years
   and his wife of 39 years, to go live down the road.
   Only five short miles separate him from his past,
   much of what he has already forgotten.
   But not his home or his wife, he still remembers them.

It is not his decision but he goes willingly like the good
   child he has become.
   And I feel like a monster that has ripped him from the
   last vestiges of his identity,
   conned him into a situation he would not have chosen.
   But choices ran out; I am running out.

Today I am losing my husband, along with a shared
   history and a life full of memories.
   Only five short miles will separate us from what was
   once our life together.

each day

Each day I travel the five miles that now separates us
   from a life we once shared.
   Sometimes for lunch, sometimes for dinner, sometimes
   just for a quick visit, but always each and every day.
   Five miles isn't far, but it seems miles away.
   So strange is this routine—shouldn't I be doing this
   with my parents, not my husband?

A thought that runs through my head as I walk down
   the hall to his room.
   Neither surprised nor glad to see me; his lack of affect
   holding strong.
   He sits in groups, not really there, but glad in some
   way to not be alone, or so it seems.

He eats dinner with great relish, thrilled to always have
seconds, but baths are still a bone of contention.
His room is decorated with favorite pictures and
mementos, but he seems not to notice.

It appears he has adjusted or is it wishful thinking?
I cannot penetrate the silence that covers him like a
protective shroud.
In many ways, nothing has changed.

the other woman

She is blondish-gray and pretty,
petite and very demure, this woman my husband has
taken up with.
They sit together on the living room couch holding
hands.
She is 80ish to his 60ish, but neither seem to notice,
nor care.
She picks the lint off his sweater, smiles sweetly and
then returns to staring straight ahead, matching his
body language.

They look like statues of lovers or more like mother and
son, now immortalized on the couch.
But when I want to take him away, she protests,
holding onto his hand with great fierceness.
I assure her, I will only borrow him for a short time,
and then return him back to her.

With trusting eyes, she relinquishes his hand,
this sweet lady who now protects and loves my husband.
This sweet lady who has become "the other woman."
This sweet lady that I now love, too.

it never stops

My elderly father, now 92, is not doing well.
   I noticed at his 92nd birthday he had slowed down
   considerably and slept more, but after all he was 92.
   But what I thought was age related, turns out not
   to be.

He needs cardiac surgery and his prostate cancer is
   moving on.
   My father, who prides himself on his independence, has
   requested I come for his surgery. This is a man who
   asks little of his family.
   It seems only I will do, not my brother. After all, this is
   woman's work.
   I am more than willing to go, but what I did not know
   then is this will be just the first of many trips to Florida.

I arrive, see him through surgery, and it is not till I am
   alone with my mother that I understand why he has
   slowed down, why he sleeps so much ... my mother has
   become even more demanding in her elderly years, if
   that is possible.

I return many times before his death, two years later.
   Now totally alone with my mother, I realize what I did
   not then ... her demandingness that I took for granted
   is dementia.

The plane trips increase.
   Luckily, my husband does not notice, does not care.
   Doctors to meet with, treatment plans to discuss,
   assisted living to pick out, followed later by a nursing
   home, and eventually Hospice to be called.

Six months following my husband's death, my mother dies.
Very soon after that my mother-in-law needs to move
to a nursing home in Maine.

My caregiving never stops. But something new has
happened out of necessity—I have learned how to set
boundaries, juggle multiple demands, and take care of
myself.

touch

A small touch—innocent enough—has jolted me back
to reality, back to moments long forgotten.

I am balancing precariously on the moving sidewalk
at the airport, each side of me weighed down with
a carry-on.

From behind me, a male hand reaches out and
steadies my back.

Surprised by the gesture, I turn around and thank him.

He smiles and goes his way, never knowing how his
kindness reunited me with long buried longings.

visits

My visits to my husband continue; we have developed
a routine.
I come into his room and greet him; he seems to know
me, like a familiar person from the past.
We sit, he stares straight ahead.
I talk, he stares straight ahead.
We walk the halls in unison, going no place in particular.
I take him to participate in an activity ... he does so
willingly, staring straight ahead.
We share a meal ... he eats, staring straight ahead.
We listen to music; he taps his feet staring straight ahead.
I share photos of the grandchildren; he stares without
recognition.

I say good-bye and I will see him tomorrow; there is no
reaction as he stares straight ahead.

intervention

My son sits me down in the kitchen, for what I assume
will be a chat.
"How are things going, Mom? Are you taking care of
yourself and finding time for you? he inquires."

But it is not our usual chat; it is an intervention.
I can hardly believe my ears as he voices his concern
I am drinking far too much wine.
How can that be?
What's wrong with a glass or maybe two, or even
three, if it's a really difficult day?
After all, this is my main coping mechanism,
my favorite part of the day when my worries and
concerns just float away.
Aren't I owed that?

But he does not see it that way, and I know in my heart,
   I am drinking too much.
   It makes my life so much easier, so much better I think,
   but I do not voice it and I know he is right.

should have known better

Almost a year into my new freedom, I have grown
   restless, tired of being alone.
   Suddenly the house is too quiet, and no longer a
   sanctuary.
   A new idea arises, and I add on a part-time job on
   weekends to my weekly four-day consulting job.
   This, along with visiting, and now I will never have a
   moment to myself.
   I like it. No time to think, no time to be lonely, no time
   to fear the future.

All is well for the next six months, till I reach the point
   of burnout.
   I should have remembered the widow from Boston
   who warned me of this, who spoke of doing the same
   until she landed in the hospital.
   Time for me to quiet down and face what needs to be
   faced.

new behaviors

Suddenly, seemingly out of nowhere, new behaviors
have begun.
Strange behaviors that are foreign to him and what he
was before.
Behaviors that make no sense, and beg the questions:
"Where did you come from and what are you about?"
My husband has become recalcitrant, obstreperous, a
real behavior problem.
Urinating in the potted plants, defecating in the
hallways, not obeying staff.

At first it was overlooked, hoping it would disappear.
But no such luck, and I am left with the thought—
how much longer will they keep him?
A question which was answered almost immediately.
It seems they would like me to bring in a caregiver,
but I am already at my financial limit.
Months pass and slowly his behavior returns to what
it was. Crisis passed.

Two years into the stay, we have hit another crisis;
he is falling all the time, resulting in trips to the ER.
They cannot keep him any longer and deem him
nursing home material, the cost of which I cannot
afford, nor do I wish to assign him to such a fate.

It is time to move for both of us.
I have found an assisted living facility that will keep
him in spite of his behaviors.
My mind is made up and I will take him, even if it is
across the country.
Even if our neurologist says, "You can't take him on
a plane to California. It would never work."
"Watch me" is my reply.

If I have learned one thing with this disease, it is to trust
my intuition.

So we are off to another assisted living memory unit
situation in California, new behaviors and all.

We are off to be near his son, which puts a smile on his
otherwise vacant face.

no way to be remembered

Torn between the needs of my father and husband,
somedays I don't know which way to turn.

My father's illness is progressing as is my husband's.

My father needs me now, my husband will have to wait.

I arrive not quite sure what this visit will entail, but I
soon find out.

His pain has increased, his strength has declined but all
that is on his mind is an enema.

No nurse in sight, the minutes, hours pass by.

Calls are made but no nurse in sight.

Someone has to give the enema.

For sure it's not going to be my mother; she wants to
go shopping.

It's not going to be my brother; he's not into things
like that.

I pour myself a glass of wine, glove up and do what
needs to be done.

Not a memory I cherish and now I understand why my
therapist says I should not change my husband's diapers.

No one should be remembered this way.

father

The plane from JFK picks up tailwinds on its flight to
Tampa, ensuring an early arrival, when every minute
counts.

I pray that my father will hold on so I can get there in
time to say good-bye.

Out of nowhere, he suddenly worsened and end was
in sight.

Each moment passes in slow agony but I make it in
time to spend his last hours with him.

He dies a beautiful, peaceful death.

He has passed before my husband,
almost like a practice run for me.

I am losing the two most important men in my life.

Two years into the stay, we
have hit another crisis; he is
falling all the time, resulting
in trips to the ER.

plane ride

He is packed up and ready to go. Double diapered,
double medicated, fed, and ready for a nonstop flight
from NYC to San Diego.
We board the plane, strangers giving us wide berth
and understanding looks.
All goes well till the pilot announces a stop in Utah; it
seems we are low on fuel due to bad weather conditions.
What was to be nonstop has now added hours to the
journey.

I pray he continues to sleep, the medication does not
wear off and the diapers hold out.
Once again airborne, we are almost there.
We are met in San Diego with a wheelchair but he
refuses to cooperate, dragging his feet and making
the process difficult. Clearly the meds have worn off.
I pray the diapers are still good.

Finally we arrive at the new assisted living memory unit,
meet with staff, and settle in.
None of this makes an impression on him and I wonder
if he even knows this is a different place.
He is thrilled to see his son, but utters no words.
As we unpack, a resident wanders in and out of his
room asking each time, "Have you seen my husband?"
My husband looks at my son and utters the first words
he has said in months, "Next time she comes in, ask
her to bring chips."
What a wonderful beginning ... I knew this was the
right decision!

some days

My life these days is divided between my husband and
my mother.
One near, one far.
Decisions to be made on their behalf,
doctors' appointments to ensure continuity of care,
visits to keep their spirits up and let them know they
are not alone.

This is what makes up my days.
Some days I feel split in half.
Some days I wish I were a twin.
Some days I am not sure where I am supposed to be.
Long distance caregiving is totally different from
caregiving for my husband, where I am there and
understand what is going on.
Twice monthly visits offer much less insight. I try to
juggle both situations as best I can, but some days
I don't know whether I am coming or going.

reaction

Interesting is my reaction to family members.
My father was easy to care for:
He wanted to know the bills were taken care of,
everything was in its place,
and to assure us we would be fine.
Changed not a bit, just tired and ready to go,
he continued to be pleasant, and in charge and I was
happy to follow along.

My husband, ravaged by dementia, continued to be his
easy-going self,
wanting:
me to be there with him,
to know his family was fine,
and finally, for me to be his mother, and I was happy to
make his days the best they could be.

My mother was her difficult self to the end, wanting: to
be the center of it all, the matriarch, to be waited upon
while being demanding and mean-spirited. I gave less
than I could have.

My mother-in-law, who had every illness known to man,
just not the medical community, finally had the real thing.
The longest lasting of all, she now had dementia.
Now ensconced in California, and exhausted from trips
to Florida for my parents, I became the true version of
long-distance caregiver.
Conversations over the phone filled my days,
always early mornings as no one could seem to
remember the time difference.

She had never been easy and she got the least of my
caregiving ways.

adjustment

The move to California turned out to be the right one.

I took a gamble, went against conventional wisdom by following my intuition and I was right.

No more urinating in potted plants or other undesirable acts.

He is happy, he is smiling, he's even talking a little bit; he is more like himself.

It's as if he finally feels at home.

honeymoons don't last forever

The honeymoon lasted 18 months or 558 days, give or take a few.

And what a honeymoon it was.

My husband acclimated well to his new environment, adjusted to the rhythms of life there, enjoyed the activities and mealtimes.

But best of all, he loved seeing his son, who stopped by often on his way to work.

And then there was the new girlfriend; age appropriate this time.

She pulled him along everywhere she went and he happily followed.

No more sitting on the couch.

No more snoozing the day away.

No more staring straight ahead.

Life is good!

And good it remained for 18 months.

No recalcitrant behavior.

No more urinating in potted plants.

Now his days are filled with a semblance of a life lost.

He has found equilibrium, and a new way of being.

All was good until the inevitable decline begins.

This time more steep, more treacherous, more rapid than previous declines.

CHAPTER 16

Hospice and Final Days

Hospice helps one to face the reality of the end, to not feel so alone in the process, and to aid in the decisions that need to be made.

The decision to call Hospice in is not an easy choice as it marks the end of the journey. My reluctance to set Hospice up evoked memories of when I had to call Hospice in for my father. He looked me straight in the eye and asked if he was dying. No such problem with my husband, who has been unaware for years.

But I am aware and full of mixed emotions. On one hand, I wanted his suffering to be ended. He could barely walk at this point, ate very little, had gone from 165 to 117 pounds, and was wasting away more each day.

California has recently put assisted suicide in place, but I am sure it is still a life-wrenching decision to make and could cause much anguish among family members. But if I have a dementia/Alzheimer's diagnosis down the road, I want to be able to make the decision while I still can and carry out the necessary and required steps. I have had too much of this disease in my life. I do not wish to be a burden, nor be remembered this way.

> **They were there to help me through that moment.**

Hospice, while a difficult decision, turned out to be a blessing and helped guide me through difficult times. I never felt alone, even when I wanted to reverse a decision concerning medication that I had agonized over. They were there to help me through that moment. They were there at the end, making it peaceful.

Recently Dr. Barak Gaster, an internist at University of Washington School of Medicine, along with fellow colleagues, has put together a five-page document called dementia-specific advance directive to supplement the regular advance directive people use. Go to *www.dementia-directive.org* to download a copy. This has brought a sense of relief to me and is now a part of my advance directive. It has moved me away from the thought of assisted suicide, as it allows me a say in the kind of care I want, if I had Alzheimer's or dementia.

hospice

Hospice has been called in.

A decision not made lightly, and in consultation with staff and his doctor.

It seems the time has come as he now requires more care, along with a different kind of care.

The same sadness I felt when I had to call in Hospice for my father comes over me in waves.

This time I understand fully what it means and where he is headed.

Hospice helps one to face the reality of the end, to not feel so alone in the process, and to aid in the decisions that need to be made.

Hospice is a blessing at the needed time, especially when one has very little experience in that area.

I came to lean on Hospice and welcome their support.

I came to look forward to their visits, filled with explanations and reassurances.

I came to respect and appreciate their services.

I came to be thankful for their loving presence.

wonder

My husband, at least I think it is he,
   is barely recognizable these days,
   down to a mere 117 pounds,
   hunched over in the demeanor of an old man,
   walking ever so slowly down the hallway.
   Stopping now and then to stretch or take a brief nap.
   He walks with an unsteady gait.
   I wonder if he has a destination in mind.
   He walks with arms wrapped around himself.
   I wonder if he misses me.
   He walks grinding his teeth incessantly.
   I wonder what demons possess him.
   Sometimes he walks arm in arm with me.
   I wonder if he even knows I am here.
   My husband is now a shell of his former self.
   I wonder where he has gone.

go away

Go away death,
  visit someone else.
  I am tired of you, weary from your presence.
  First you took our beloved dog, far too early.
  Then my father when I needed him most.
  My mother is on hospice and my husband is
  dying a slow death.
  Now you've put your claim on my best friend's
  husband.
  And if that isn't enough, you are circling
  another friend.

Go away death.
  You are not welcome.
  Take your decay.
  Take your darkness.
  Take your sadness and go away.

witness

Nothing in life prepares one to be a witness to the slow
  decline of another,
  the agonizing loss of mind,
  the horrific decay of body.
  This disease is cruel beyond all description.
  Final Stage is the most difficult of all.
  A time when friends and family visit less often;
  "I just want to remember him as he was," the response
  most often given.

Do they think I want any different?
  Do they think I have been given superpowers to stay
  the course?
  The questions and answers are irrelevant....
  I may not have superpowers, but I have been given the
  grace and fortitude to see it through.
  And for that, I am eternally grateful.

long

Final Stage can often be the longest stage of all, that's
   what the books say, that's what the experts say.
   But this long?
   This is beyond endurable.
   He has no life now, and yet he goes on to greet
   another day, not even knowing it has arrived.
   It's like being stuck at a railroad crossing with a long
   train approaching.
   It's like a game with no tie breaker.
   It's like an endless wave.
   He exists in his own world, connected to very little
   these days.
   No games, no TV, no music.
   Even food, his great passion, has no meaning.
   He's just there and I know the man I once knew, would
   never forgive me for allowing this to happen to him.

his days

His days hold so little now.
   Not even the basics seem to interest him anymore.
   Awareness is no longer a part of his repertoire.

He seems so alone, so vulnerable and lost.
   My heart goes out to him, to protect him and keep him
   safe, but I can't reach him.
   I am his wife but he seems not to know or care.
   All I can do is be present and, sometimes, I wonder if
   he is even aware I am here?

cruel

Hasn't enough been taken away from him already?
His retirement years, his health, his grandchildren,
his family, his memory, his recognition, and eventually
his life?
How much more does this cruel disease need to steal
from him?
He is lost in a world where no one can reach him, no
one can love him, and no one can make him feel safe.
Before *Final Stage,* we still had him ... even if it was just
glimpses.
But now he is gone, except for a shell and a soul that
only he can reach.
This is the cruelest of diseases ... for those inflicted
with it and for those who much watch, unable to do
anything.

dirty little secret

A horrible little secret follows me around, but I can tell
no one.
A horrible little secret that shocks me and makes me
wonder what kind of person I am.
A horrible little secret that I know other caregivers
have had, but that makes no difference to me.
A horrible little secret that wishes him dead from his
misery and me from mine.

but years later ...

He walks banging into walls, seeming not to notice, not
to care; someday very soon, he will forget how to walk.
He sleeps curled up in a ball in front of the elevator.
I wonder if he is planning his escape; someday very
soon he will never leave his bed.

He seems not to know me nor care I am there until
the moment I see a small glimmer in his eye; someday
very soon, he will no longer know who I am—not even
a glimmer.

So painful to see him this way, stripped down to bare
basics, as if he never was a person.

But years later, I am glad I did what I did, went when I
did not want to.

The grandchildren visit and I see fear on the little one's
face as she watches him.

I worry this will scar her, but years later she tells me
lovely stories about her visit and I fill in with details
she never got to know.

Sometimes, I feel as if I don't know him; he is a stranger
I visit.

So hard is it to reconnect with the once vital person I
knew. The once loving husband I had.

But years later, those memories will return, and I will
find him again as he once was.

It is not easy staying the course and I understand why
some people bolt, having wanted to myself on many
an occasion.

But years later I will be so thankful I stayed the course
'till the end.

*At the beginning, in the blur of adapting, our neurologist told
me he wanted me to have no regrets at the end. It was so far
away then; I could not appreciate his advice. But years later,
I am so grateful, so very, very grateful for his sage advice.*

the christmas gift

Christmas has arrived once again.
  Where does the time go?
  We celebrate this Christmas Eve by walking the almost
  deserted halls, a pastime now very familiar to both of us.
  Sometimes I wonder how many miles we've logged on
  our little journey together.

To break the monotony of this repetitious task,
  I ask a question, not expecting an answer from a man
  who has not spoken in months.
  "Do you know who I am?" I ask.
  And to my great surprise he replies, "The love of my life."
  Those were the last words he ever spoke to me and
  the best Christmas present he ever gave me.

anticipatory grief

Anticipatory grief is now moving toward grief as he
  moves closer and closer to the end of his journey.
  Increasingly frail, weakened with no appetite and
  sleeping constantly, no longer aimlessly walking the
  halls, I know he is preparing to leave this world and
  move on.
  I feel the shift in my attitude and of those around me.
  There is a sadness mixed with relief as the days
  stretch on.

decision

Pneumonia has set in and after many consultations with
   the nurse, I have decided not to treat it but, instead,
   see where it goes.
   Not an easy decision and reached with much anguish
   and thought.
   He had declined markedly before the pneumonia—
   lost weight, slept most of the time, wandered the
   hallway bumping into walls, and remained almost
   comatose.
   Without medications, his condition is worsening and
   I am feeling badly, and confused.

I call the nurse, telling her I have changed my mind, and
   she reminds me of our past conversations, of what he
   would have wanted, and of what it will be like for him
   going forward, if we treat him.

I thank her for the support and kindness and tell her
   I am sticking with my original decision—saddened as
   I am but supported by the belief he never would have
   wanted to live in his present condition.
   Another angel in my life.

> **Without medications,
> his condition is worsening
> and I am feeling badly,
> and confused.**

last breath

The vigil, the countdown, the death march, the final
hours or whatever it is called has now begun.
We are gathered—his family—in silence around his bed.
There are no words, except "I love you," and "You can
go when you are ready," to utter, to share.

We knew this day would come; we even wished it to
come at times, but we always thought it would be
another day, another time.

We thought we were prepared, but that was a
misconception once reality with its finality arrived.
Now we will no longer see him or be with him, only in
our hearts, only in our memories.

We hold our breath as his breathing slows down,
afraid it will be his last breath.
But it is not, and he goes on.

We worry he is in pain and suffering, but the Hospice
nurse assures us he is not. She is monitoring the
situation all along.

We are grateful that in the end, she can do for him what
we cannot, so we wait, dreading that final moment,
that final breath that will change the structure of our
family forever.

**We knew this day would come;
we even wished it to come at times,
but we always thought it would be
another day, another time.**

reminders

Breathe.
Embrace your feelings, don't run from them,
don't hang on so tightly,
remember you are strong but cry when you feel like it,
acknowledge that this is out of your hands.
Know that he will be at peace soon, freed from this
hideous disease,
and know that you can and will go on.

These are the reminders, I tell myself, when I think I can't
do this one more moment.
These are the reminders I tell myself, when life without
him seems impossible.

darkness

My days have been filled with a new kind of darkness
as we edge slowly to the end of this journey.
There is a sadness that comes with the inevitable,
when nothing more can be done, and the slow death
march has begun in earnest.
A time when all we can do is be present for him
and for ourselves, and not give into the desire to run
and hide.
And trust that lightness will return to him and our
family when the time is right.

all I can do

All I can do is stare straight ahead.

All I can do is not move.

All I can do is stay locked in my thoughts.

I have become my husband ... blocked off and shut
down, as if he left his body and I now inhabit it.
None of it makes sense, even though I knew it was
inevitable, even though I was prepared.
But you are never prepared for the last breath
someone takes.
Nothing can prepare you for the finality of it.

So I stare straight ahead.

So I don't move.

So I stay locked in my thoughts, waiting for the shock
to wear off.

stopped

His breathing has stopped.

The room has become eerily silent.
A feeling of being suspended, not connected has
overcome me.
We are frozen, my family and I: no one moves for what
seems like an eternity.
Is this the end we all waited for of which
part of me never believed would happen?
My mind can't seem to reconcile what has just occurred.
Where is the answer to my question?

Surely, this is not the end.

I walk out of the room to do something I must do at the nurse's station. What is it I must do?

I must be sleep walking. Maybe they will know. Maybe they will have answers for my questions. Nothing feels real anymore.

In a fog, I make it back to the nearby condo I am renting and sit in a stupor on the couch.

My daughter stares at me in a parallel stupor.

My son looks shell-shocked.

This can't be happening continues to run through my mind, like an intrusive melody that will not stop.

"This is the end. This is the best thing that could have happened to my husband," I tell myself.

But suddenly, I am not so sure of anything.

AFTERMATH

The aftermath is different for each and every caregiver and plays out in a way that is unique to him/her. For me, the first few months were a complete blur. By the end of the first year, I was on steadier ground and ready to start looking at my life again. So much work has to be done during this time period—wills, Social Security, transfer of assets—the list goes on forever. Just at a time when you think it is all over, you find a flurry of activities that need your attention.

Around the six month mark I started to venture out and took a few short trips with girlfriends. One outing in particular stands out.... We visited an art gallery and then went into the next room where a small group of college students were giving a concert. Suddenly, I felt tears rolling down my face; my senses, so long deprived, were overwhelmed. Until that point, I hadn't realized the full magnitude of the isolation that had surrounded my life.

Slowly I forged ahead in the world and tentatively became use to my new life. My home in Connecticut seemed very lonely and full of memories that were both soothing and disconcerting at the same time. I did not want to live the rest of my life with only memories to sustain me. I also did not want to lead the same suburban life I had always lived.

Here was an opportunity to try a different kind of life, and I reached back into my past and connected with my desire to live near the beach. This is what prompted my permanent move to California and an added bonus, it was nice to be near my son and his family. I now had an opportunity to be me, not the widow I was in Connecticut.

I hadn't realized the full magnitude of the isolation that had surrounded my life.

days

Days pass slowly, some slower than others.
Some days pass in a blur of activity.
Friends come and go bringing condolences.
Lawyers and CPAs are busy doing what they do best.
Family has come and gone, assuring me all along I will
be fine.
It feels like an out-of-body experience; not quite real,
not happening to me.
But it is, and he is gone.
Everybody agrees it is best for him, best for me.
Sentiments I once shared, but not now.
Suddenly I am immobilized, frozen in the past.
This is not real; this is not happening.

grief

Grief wraps around me like a coat two sizes too big.
Loneliness surrounds my heart leaving room for
nothing else.
Despair sits on my shoulders weighing me down.
Sadness is etched on my face making it unfamiliar to
me in the mirror.
Gone is the bounce in my step,
the lilt in my voice.
I have become older than my chronological years,
having traveled to places so foreign.
Now I am returning from an unplanned journey.
Just not to the life I had or the person I was.

thawing out

Thawing out, that is what I am doing.
    Slowly, day by day, part by part, I am getting myself
    back, gaining equilibrium, and focusing on my future.
    I wish this process would move faster, but I am glad it
    is moving.

This loss, more monumental than any before, will always be
    with me, and has now become a part of who I now am.
    This loss—so strong, so unrelenting—will diminish in
    time I trust, but I know it will never go away.
    Tears flow when least expected, but laughter now
    comes at the most unexpected times.
    Thawing out takes time, making room for the new life
    to come.

**But a new life awaits, so
finally I find the words to
talk—about my new life.**

gift

I sit in the psychologist's office, the one who I have seen
over the course of my husband's illness.
We meet now to keep me on course and to help me
cope with the inevitable that has come.
We meet so I can continue to work on the ongoing
issues of grief.
My therapist begins as he always does, inquiring how I
have been, but I am in no mood for small talk.
So stunned by the reality of it, the finality,
I want to shout out, "My life is over."
But I already know what he would say, so I remain
silent with my whirling thoughts.

In many ways my life is over ... the life I have known and
lived for all these years.
But a new life awaits, so finally I find the words to
talk—about my new life, the uncertainties I face,
my new role of widow, along with the numerous
decisions to be made.

We talk, my therapist and I, as we have in the past in
preparation for this moment.
We talk now with a new sense of earnestness and
direction, about the process of letting go of yesterday,
greeting today, and the days that follow,
about being present in the moment,
about starting my new life, now that the time has
arrived.

This is what my husband would have wanted.

This is my final gift to him.

CHAPTER 17

Finding Tomorrow and New Beginnings

Finding your tomorrow is not an easy task after years of caregiving and caregiver has become one's identity. It entails preparation, thought, decision making, and ability to forge a new identity. Preparation for tomorrow is best started at the beginning, when all that is required is a simple planting of the seed. Simple, because there is not much time in *Beginning Stage* to think about anything other than diagnosis and the changes it brings. But the process begins here, even it is just a random thought tucked away in the back of your mind.

By *Middle Stage,* most caregivers have joined a support group and it is there, where the discussion of one's tomorrow is discussed, along with many other topics. The process can be as simple as, afterwards, do I want to stay in the same home or do I want to move closer to my children? Or, am I ready for an independent or assisted living facility? These are the kick-start questions that start to point caregivers toward tomorrow.

By *Final Stage*, plans must be in place, even if only tentative, because when death arrives, it is followed by the mourning process, leaving one less open or available to making changes; just at the time when changes are being called upon to be made.

There is an old rule of thumb to do nothing big in the way of change the first year following a death of a loved one, but this rule does not exempt anyone from planning and laying the groundwork for tomorrow.

So how do you find your tomorrow? Start by giving yourself quiet moments to remember who you were before caregiving. This is accomplished by focusing on your former dreams, your likes and dislikes, things which gave you pleasure, and your values. This will help you to get back in touch with parts of yourself that have been lost or put on the back shelf during your caregiving years. I found a combination of walks on the beach and meditation were helpful to quiet the mind and focus.

Throughout my caregiving journey, I always knew I wanted to live near the ocean someday, and I started to collect objects that reflected that longing. Once on an outing with my girlfriends, I purchased a painting of four women at the beach, even though I had nowhere to put it. My friends thought I was crazy and encouraged me to not purchase it. Today it hangs happily in my house by the beach. In my quest for my future, I ordered a painting of a small home with a red door that opened to a beach view, from a catalogue. When it arrived, I hung it on the wall in my bedroom to remind me I did have a future. Years later when I moved to San Diego, I hung it in my front hallway, and it was not until months later, I realized my new beach home also had a red front door. There is power in putting your wishes and desires out to God, the universe, or whatever you believe in.

Finding tomorrow means, along the way, you take time for yourself. As all caregivers know, that is almost an impossibility, but respites or short visits to friends and family are a great help. For years you have been taking care of someone else, now it's your turn to take care of yourself.

After my husband died, I took almost a year off to just think and process what I had been through. I began preparations to sell my Connecticut home and move to California. That was enough for me to do as I found I didn't have the energy or desire to do much else, and I was content to just "be" and revel in the quietness of my life.

Much of the grieving process had occurred over the years before as I mourned each new loss along the way; this is defined as anticipatory grieving and is an inevitable part of the disease and a caregiver's life. Not that there wasn't grieving still left to do, it was just much of it had been accomplished over the course of the disease. After a year, I was ready to move on and discover what life held. I still have moments, special times, smells, that take me back and bring sadness, but nothing to the degree I had before. Learning to let go, as life demands, has become part of my repertoire.

The question of dating and when it is appropriate to begin, was a question often raised in my support group. Some people started when their spouse was placed in an assisted living or nursing home. Others waited till after the end came, and then wrestled with what is the appropriate time to pass. There is no rule or etiquette around this decision and the reality that many of us are already in our declining years, impacts the decision. Going on a few dates after my husband died, I found the experience exciting, depressing, hysterically funny, and a pain in the rear. I knew I never wanted to marry; afraid I would end up being a caregiver again, even though I was well aware it might be me who needed caregiving. This, however, did not change my decision. I have known others who have married and are delightfully happy, and those who remained single and the same can be said of them. It is a wonderful time in our lives when we are free of "must do's" or rigid game plans.

don't worry

I have cocooned, safe in my house, nestled away from
the world.

I may not seem busy to others ... lolling around all day,
reading books, and turning down invitations.

But this is what I need ... time and distance from
the world.

Time where my head can stop spinning, my heart stop
pounding, and days belong just to me.

For, unbeknownst to you, I am busy replenishing my soul,
finding my former self, reconciling the past and the
future, while re-inventing myself.

Each day I am pointed closer to tomorrow.

One day my metamorphosis will be complete, so you
need not worry about me.

famous bunny

I was like the proverbial Energizer Bunny that kept going
and going and going.

"Still Going" was his slogan, along with a fit pink body
and trademark sunglasses, marching to his own drum,
making him a superstar.

No superstar am I, no pink body do I have, but the
trademark sunglasses and marching to our own drum
we have in common.

So, like the pink bunny, I kept going and going and
going, over the days, over the weeks, over the months,
over the years.

But, unlike the pink bunny, I couldn't keep it up.

My battery depleted, my spirit wore down, with barely
enough juice left to see me through.

Now today, trademark sunglasses in place, I am
recharging my battery, finding myself, and happily
marching to my own drum.

And best of all, I am still going!

Encore

Love maybe lovelier the second time around, but I can tell you this for sure, Alzheimer's is not. A few years after the death of my husband, and having dated a few men that would drive any woman to the nunnery, I met a lovely widowed gentleman. We had a lot in common: We liked trying new restaurants out, hanging out at the beach, going to the theater, and traveling to new and exciting places.

We had a wonderful three years together until I begun to see signs of memory loss, which I convinced myself I noticed only because I was overly sensitive to the issue. There it was in full bloom denial— wouldn't you have thought I would have learned the first time around? I so wanted this relationship to work that I chose to overlook the signs and I told myself all was fine. As we all know too well, there comes a time when signs cannot be overlooked. It felt like déjà vu again as friends assured me he was fine, his daughters saw no issues, and the neurologist I took him to, thought it was MCI, and not to worry. It was only after repeated requests on my part, that he ordered a four hour neurological test. This resulted in a mid-stage diagnosis and a gracious, to his credit, apology.

So the process began once again, but at a faster pace. In California, when one is diagnosed with Alzheimer's or dementia, the state takes away all driving privileges; a process that impacts every aspect of one's life. While he didn't live full time with me, he was there very often. Without a drivers license, he was no longer able to make the thirty mile trek that separated us. Suddenly, he was with me full time and it wasn't long before old habits and feelings began to return. I had become a full time caregiver as I took him to doctors, helped with errands, and the numerous other activities that go on.

A year into this my doctor told me I had a mild case of post traumatic stress disorder or better known as PTSD. I later went on to develop AFib, as his symptoms and behaviors increased and my energy and patience were drained. All this occurred while I was helping him sell his home, find an assisted living, and get him moved in, proving to be much harder the second time around. I knew without a doubt, I could not take on an encore. I was prepared to help out, get him set, and continue to have him in my life, but it would be on my terms. He was a wonderful companion, but he was not my husband.

Around this time a good friend took me aside and inquired if I was okay because she thought I seemed different. My daughter, a little while later, reported to me that my grand-daughter, who is my biggest advocate, didn't think I was as much fun and was worried about me. Once again, it took someone else to help me see what I could not see myself ... I was getting worn out.

The young neuropsychologist, when finished delivering test results, took me aside and told me to not become the one responsible, as families sometimes find it easier to let the girlfriend or second wife do it all while they bow out. I know it sounds sappy or California woo-woo, but I believe there are angels along our way to guide and support us. I was so thankful for her concern and kindness for my well-being. Sometimes you just need to hear it from someone else.

I cared deeply for this man, knew I would miss his companionship, was well aware of the lack of eligible men in my age bracket, but this I knew for sure … there would be no encore for me. I see him occasionally, take him to lunch or an outing with friends, but the nature of the relationship has changed, and as this book went to press, he has continued to decline with the disease.

how did this happen?

How did this happen?
   I told myself I'd never be a caregiver again.
   I was done...end of story.
   How did this happen?
   Here I am a caregiver again.
   When I met him he was fun and full of adventure.
   We laughed, we traveled, we enjoyed the thrill of the
   newness and I chose, knowing better
   to overlook the signs.
   Lonely, tired of being alone, it was easier to go along

with the promise of tomorrow.
But tomorrow has arrived and the promise is not what
I thought it would be.

encore

Somedays I can hardly tell the difference …
is it then or now?
Who are you?

I seem not to know, calling you by husband's name,
confusing you with him in my dreams.
This is déjà vu, this is Groundhog Day, and this is all
too familiar.
I open the window, you close it.
I put something away, you put it in a place never to be
seen again.
I sit down to do something, you suddenly need me.
I am responsible for your day, my day has disappeared.
I thought the play had ended, the curtain brought down.
But this feels like an Encore, and a very long one at that.

saving me, at last

Sadness,
guilt,
disappointment,
relief.
An array of emotions, evoked by fact that I could no
longer take care of my companion, overtook me.
Not my husband,
not my family,
not really my responsibility.
This is what I told myself.

But, nonetheless, a wonderful companion of many
years and someone I cared for.
Still, I am not as young as I once was,
with more years behind me, than ahead.
Now is the time to take care of myself.
Now it the time to do what I want to do.
Now is the time to make up for those lost years.
Things I tell myself, things my children tell me.
As Mary Oliver, the poet, so eloquently put it in her
poem, "The Journey:"
I was determined to save the only life I could save.
And save my life. I did.

TODAY

So what am I doing now that my caregiver days are behind
me? I am happy to be on my own, and be busy with family
and grandchildren, going to outings, traveling with girlfriends, and just simply enjoying life in "Paradise," as San
Diego is often referred to. It would be lovely to have a man
in my life, but no longer a necessity. I have learned how to
be alone and not lonely. I have willingly given up years to
caregiving, and now this is my time and I am going to
enjoy it. I am at peace with all that has gone before and I
am looking forward to tomorrow.

So how will your tomorrow look? That pretty much depends
on how much effort you want to put into it. Give yourself a
rest before you start in, but gather your thoughts along the

way, and when you are ready to start, things will begin to fall into place. Remember to not let anyone tell you what you should do. You have come through a long journey, and your intuition, strength, and courage that carried and supported you so far will serve you well going forward. Start sooner than later to Point Yourself toward Tomorrow. There is life after caregiving, but it is a life that must be found and created by you.

remember

You have returned in dreams but, most importantly, in my memories.

I remember you now, as you were before this horrible disease took hold and ravished you.

I remember you now that time has passed and caregiving no longer consumes my days.

I remember who you were.

I remember my husband.

I remember my children's father.

I remember my grandchildren's grandfather.

I remember our life together.

I remember now with love and gratitude.

It is so good to have you back.

inquiring minds want to know

People ask, "How you are doing now that it's over?"

And my reply is "Good enough."

Years ago, when overwhelmed by caregiving
responsibilities, and trying desperately to be the best
I could, I discovered the concept "good enough."

And since that moment, my outlook changed.

Most caregivers think they didn't do enough.

Didn't try hard enough,

didn't last as long as they should have,

but, that is simply not true.

Most caregivers have gone way beyond the expected,
sacrificed more than humanly possible, and endured
what many are not capable of.

And so it is in my life now.

It's not the life I planned,

not the retirement I dreamed of,

but it's good enough, and sometimes even more.

question

Will you remarry?

A question often asked.

More so when I had a companion, but even now.

"No," is the answer I hold steadfastly to, even
knowing never to say no.

This is my time.

I traded in the family home with all its wonderful
memories, for a tiny condo by the ocean.

I downsized my life, prioritized, and re-invented myself,
now that the role of wife is no longer mine and
the title widow much too depressing.

Today I lead a simpler life, a "good enough" life
with time, at last, for me.

And for all of that, I am immensely grateful.

so you want to know

So many questions people ask … so many things people
want to know.
I understand, I once was in that place, too.
I thought their answers would guide me, give me
direction … and they did.
But I also learned to look to myself for answers that
would fit me, as you will also.

What have you learned?
To be present by letting go of what I thought would
happen and live, instead, in what is happening.

Has it changed you?
Yes, I am not the same person I was at the beginning of
the journey. I like to think I am more compassionate and
aware of the life plight of others, along with being more
receptive and giving.

What would you tell others?
Trust your instincts, listen to your heart as well as your
head, be kind to yourself by making room for yourself,
and, above all, know you will be fine.

Do you have any regrets?
Yes, I have regrets but not many and regrets are just a
waste of today.

How did you make it through?
One day at a time, one foot in front of the other, and by
showing up, even when I didn't want to.

Are you angry or upset that your life has been rearranged?
Why me? has become Why not me?
What was the most valuable lesson you learned?
If I could tell caregivers only ONE thing, it would be …
don't make this journey alone. Reach out and ask for
help and be receptive and open to accepting it. This is a
gift to you and a gift to those who want to help.

my life now

My life is different now—so different from how I once
envisioned it.

Once being a long time ago before the diagnosis and
ravages of Alzheimer's.

A time so long ago, I can barely remember it or the
woman I was then.

Before necessity dictated my life be rearranged, before
retirement was drastically altered,

before widow became my designation.

But, still it is not a bad life, just a different life.

I am here—a testimonial to the human spirit.

Having made adjustments, altered attitudes, loved and
supported my husband through the final days.

I am ready for my new life.

story

Our story, our journey is over and finished or so it seems,
   but is it ever?
   I think not.
   My husband will live on in the memories of:
   me,
   his children,
   his grandchildren,
   his friends,
   his coworkers,
   and those who read this book.
   In the shiny pennies we find at just the right time,
   letting us know he is watching over us.

His life was too short
   and we often wonder why,
   but there is no answer, so we choose acceptance.
   We shall move forward, pointed toward tomorrow,
   forever changed:
   humbler,
   kinder,
   wiser,
   taking nothing for granted,
   grateful to have been blessed with the spirit and
   tenacity to stay the course,
   and saying a prayer each night, for those who now
   go after us.

after thought

I have been asked by,
  well-wishers, friends, strangers,
  people afflicted with the disease,
  even family,
  why I would go public with our story?
  Why am I so involved with the Alzheimer's Association?
  Why would I write a book sharing my innermost feelings?
  Why do I lecture on the subject?
  Why did we agree to appear on CBS?
  Why now that he has passed on, do I not just forget all
  about it and simply enjoy myself?

I ponder these questions and hope they are asked out
  of simple curiosity, and not with a hidden message or
  innuendo.

I have no reply except:
  until you are dealing with a disease so feared,
  people don't want to hear or speak about it,
  a disease that Medicare places restrictions on, and the
  one benefit needed, custodial long-term nursing home
  care, is not covered,
  until you fear that there is a possibility that your
  children could share such a similar fate,
  until you have sat through one too many jokes about
  Alzheimer's or senior moments,
  until you have experienced the pain of people
  distancing themselves,
  until you truly understand the tsunami-type growth
  predicted for this disease,
  and have seen the figures that make it now the most
  expensive and feared disease in the country,
  only then will you understand why.

What I can tell you is:
  this is not a disease to be ashamed of,
  this is not a disease to be hidden away,
  and this is not a disease to leave families to suffer
  in silence or deplete their financial and emotional
  resources.

This is a disease that needs to be understood, not feared.
  This is a disease where no longer will those afflicted,
  be marginalized or forgotten.
  This is a disease that must marshal Congress for more
  money for research and programs.
  And one of the ways to accomplish this is to go public
  with your story,
  to stand up and be counted,
  and to join in the fight for a cure.

Acknowledgements

The days, months, and even years it can take to write a book, caught me by surprise and gave me a new respect for those who write. At an authors' seminar, I offhandedly commented on how I often skipped over paragraphs, and a woman in the crowd said in a horrified tone, "How can you do that when an author labors over each written word." I later came to find out how very true that was. Writing the book is just the beginning and the most enjoyable part—then comes, editing, re-writing, formatting, and marketing. Nonetheless, it has been a labor of love, a time of great sadness revisited, a life-altering experience, and a commitment fulfilled that I made to myself to tell our story and increase awareness of this dreaded, nasty illness, along with the plight of caregivers, who are often forgotten.

Many thanks to my daughter Laura who helped me edit, caught me when I duplicated a story in another chapter, and always encouraged me to keep going.

To my son, Brian, who most of the time, overlooked my lack of computer experience, and saw me through numerous crises. I could not have done it without his expertise.

I have thanked my Healthcare Team in my book, but special thanks must go to Stephen Eliot, PhD, my therapist. He was my guiding light, source of comfort, and teacher on my long journey. I am forever grateful for the time we spent together.

To Rebecca Finkel, who soothed my never-ending angst over the placement of commas, thank you for your patience, expertise, and help. She captured the essence of my book with her cover.

To Ashlee Bratton, who took my book and website photos despite, my being an unwilling subject, you captured me perfectly.

To Judith Briles, The Book Shepherd®, it was my lucky day when I found her on the internet. Publishing is not an easy endeavor and there are many charlatans out there ready to take your money and disappear. Judith guided me through the process with her direct and honest evaluation and approach. She was able to see things, that I was not, thus bringing my book to a higher level. Plus, it was an enjoyable process to work with her.

About the Author

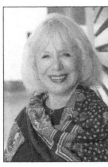

Susan Miller is a former caregiver, support group leader, lecturer and workshop presenter on the various facets of Alzheimer's for family and professional caregivers.

She is a strong advocate for caregivers —the second victim in a disease that steals something from everyone it touches. Susan has walked the walk, and knows the steps along the journey.

Her background, which includes wife, mother, school teacher, realtor, corporate trainer in both corporate America and the healthcare world, counselor, and outplacement specialist, reflects her impressive versatility.

Susan has a master's in counseling. Combining her education and work experience with her personal caregiving experience, she brings extensive expertise and wisdom to the issue of caregiving, loss, and letting go. As a national speaker, she has traveled to Washington to present on behalf of caregivers, lectured at various Alzheimer's Associations, nursing homes, and assisted living facilities.

She and her past husband were featured in a CBS three-part series on this dreaded disease.

When Susan is not speaking, you will find her in San Diego by the beach, where she and her dog, Lulu, spend hours walking and enjoying the calm the beach brings to her soul.

CareGiverBooks@gmail.com
AlzheimersCaregiverAdvocate.com
SusanGMiller22@gmail.com
760-815-0099

Working with Susan Miller

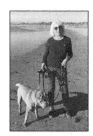

Susan speaks for a variety of groups including assisted living, nursing homes, Alzheimer's associations, pharmaceutical companies and nursing associations. Her topics include:

Up Close & Personal: my journey from beginning to end. **Bring Susan Miller** to your organization and she will provide participants with an overview of what to expect and experience throughout the Alzheimer's journey, while bringing clarity, tips, direction, and hope.

Beginning Stage: making sense of it all. **Bring Susan Miller** to your organization and she will answer the three top questions everyone asks after diagnosis, "Where do we go now, what do we do, where do we start?"

Middle Stage: a time of increased changes and responsibilities. **Bring Susan Miller** to your organization and she will help participants deal with the often overwhelming tasks and responsibilities of this stage, by offering suggestions, tips, and humor, along with her story.

Final Stage: preparing for the inevitable. **Bring Susan Miller** to your organization and she will help participants with the difficult choices of placement or in-home care, to resuscitate or not, and how to stay connected while letting go, so one can successfully navigate final stage with few regrets.

Finding Tomorrow: discovering the path to a new you. **Bring Susan Miller** to your organization and she will show caregivers YES, there is a life after caregiving, and how they can find theirs, when the time comes.

Susan Miller's exemplary journey through her husband's diagnosis and illness is inspirational and of benefit to anyone who has a loved one diagnosed with Alzheimer's disease. For those not fortunate enough to hear this outstanding speaker read her poetry, this collection of poems is the next best thing.

—Jan Mashman, MD, Associated Neurologists, Danbury, CT, retired

You spoke my thoughts, my feelings, and my yearnings at losing my spirit. Your book is the first piece of literature that pierced my heart. I have never seen a more unclouded picture of life with a beloved partner who becomes a stranger.

—Gloria Gutnes

CONNECT WITH SUSAN MILLER

CareGiverBooks@gmail.com

AlzheimersCaregiverAdvocate.com

SusanGMiller22@gmail.com

760-815-0099

Partial proceeds from sale of this book will go to Alzheimer's Association and/or Alzheimer's Research.

Made in the USA
Columbia, SC
28 May 2021

38677093R00163